THE GREA

Evelyn Lord is a local historian
College, Cambridge. She is the author of *The Hell-Fire Clubs*, *The Stuart Secret Army* and *The Knights Templar in Britain*. She is now the chair of the Cambridgeshire Association for Local History and the convenor of the Landscape and Local History Research Group. In 2019 she edited and contributed to *The Singing Milkmaids: Life in Post-Restoration Huntingdonshire*, and in 2020 compiled and contributed to *Cambridgeshire in the Archives: A Collection of Essays Celebrating Cambridgeshire Archives' New Home in Ely*.

THE GREAT PLAGUE

WHEN DEATH CAME TO CAMBRIDGE IN 1665

Evelyn Lord

YALE UNIVERSITY PRESS
NEW HAVEN AND LONDON

For information about this and other Yale University Press publications, please contact:
U.S. Office: sales.press@yale.edu   www.yalebooks.com
Europe Office: sales@yaleup.co.uk   www.yalebooks.co.uk

Set in Adobe Caslon Pro by IDSUK (DataConnection) Ltd
Printed in Great Britain by Clays Ltd, Elcograf S.p.A

Library of Congress Control Number: 2022943126

ISBN 978-0-300-17381-9 (hbk)
ISBN 978-0-300-27025-9 (pbk)

A catalogue record for this book is available from the British Library.

10 9 8 7 6 5 4 3

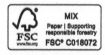

To Edward, Gabriel, Natascha and Roderick Lord, and Annice Lord, a new addition to the family since 2014, and in memory of Katie Lord with love

CONTENTS

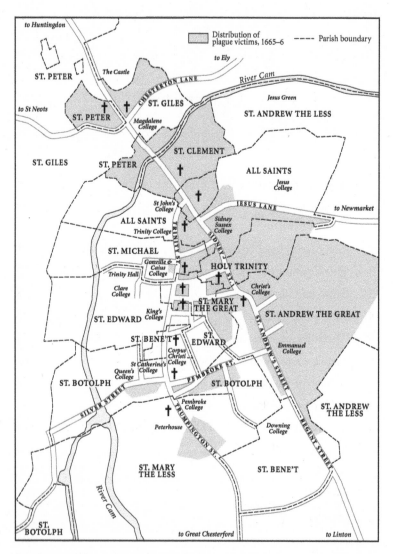

Distribution of plague victims in 1665–6. Note the unshaded areas around the colleges with the exception of Christ's College and Emmanuel.

PREFACE

THIS BOOK was written before the arrival of COVID, a modern plague. The reader will recognise similarities between the actions taken and experiences during COVID and the great plague. Sealing up infected houses in the plague has a parallel in the lockdowns of 2020, and the shortage of provisions in 1665 and 1666 as producers were reluctant to come into town is mirrored by the empty shelves in supermarkets, caused first by panic buying and then by difficulties in the supply chain in 2020. Just as in the great plague tricksters played on people's fears of infection with false claims of providing protection and cure, so in COVID criminals also played on fear by selling false vaccinations. Doubtless the reader will find other parallels from experience while reading about the seventeenth-century plague. Today we have preventative vaccinations and a growing number of anti-viral medicines to combat COVID. In the seventeenth century there was nothing like this. However, just as COVID demonstrated how friends, neighbours and the community could come together to help those isolated alone indoors without close families nearby and means of getting provisions and medicine, so in the seventeenth century friends and neighbours would have passed food and water through windows, and perhaps smuggled out uninfected children. There are no sources to tell us that this really happened but humanity suggests it did and they are the unsung heroes of history, just as COVID has resulted in the unacknowledged help of many unsung heroes of today.

In the 1990s I was the lecturer in local history at one of the newer universities. Part of the students' programme was to research and write a third-year dissertation on a subject of their own choosing. One of the mature students chose to write on a seventeenth-century village in the Peak District, matching up houses and families through probate material and other local sources. When the dissertation was completed and handed in, her husband found her in tears, and on being asked what was the matter she replied, 'They are all dead now,' 'they' being her dissertation families. When her husband pointed out that they had been dead for hundreds of years, she replied, 'But they were alive to me.'[1] This is one of the aims of local history, to bring the ordinary people of the past alive, and as Helen Cam perceptively wrote in 1944, 'the local historian starts from a present-day objective reality, whether building, boundary, name or custom; he [*sic*] holds the live end of an unbroken thread running back into the past . . .'[2] As the thread attached to 'relatively small geographical areas or communities, micro history can provide much valuable information on the macro questions of life, work and death'.[3] This book aims to follow the thread of history to Cambridge and the long hot summers of 1665 and 1666, in order to bring the people who lived and died at that time alive, and record their lives, experiences and deaths for the present day.

Over the last few years a different way of presenting history to the reader has emerged, which sheds a new perspective on the past. This tells the story through sources, but invents 'situations and dialogue, and employs techniques reminiscent of docudrama'.[4] This method, sometimes called 'faction', was used to good effect by Professor Hatcher in his book on the Black Death, and robustly defended by him in an article in *History* (January 2012). It is a method that I have used often in the past when teaching mature adult education students, by taking on the persona of a historical character for example, or by covering an event as prosaic as life in the medieval village and telling a story, but ending the session by explaining how the story was compiled and the sources used to do this. Thus, some of the scenes and descriptions in this book are imagined, but based on the sources. (The sources used for the discovery of Cambridge life in 1665 and 1666 are detailed in the Appendix.)

Why has Cambridge been chosen as the place for this exploration of the past? Cambridge in 1665 was a town settling down after the Civil War, which had caused tension between a mainly Royalist university and a mainly Parliamentarian town, and the Restoration of Charles II in 1660, which had resulted in a purge of the town's corporation and reprisals against college fellows who had supported Parliament. In 1665 the town and university looked forward to a settled and economically fruitful existence in which the town's feasts and fairs could be celebrated, and couples could marry and raise children in peace, but over this optimism hung the spectre of the plague.

The effect of the great plague of 1665 and 1666 on London is well known. Many books have been written about it, most of them based on the Bills of Mortality, which listed the numbers of people who died each week, and how many of these died from plague. Cambridge issued Bills of Mortality as well, and although the percentage of plague deaths was high, Cambridge was much smaller than London, so that by using other sources it is possible to identify where the plague victims lived and to reconstruct their lives, and so produce an intimate picture of Cambridge in a time of crisis.

Seventeenth-century Cambridge was a town of overlapping communities that symbiotically meshed together: the colleges and the university, the town corporation, shopkeepers, craftsmen, labourers and the poor. This allows for the examination of many different people's experience of the plague; for example, that of the college fellow and the college servant, a wealthy alderman and an impoverished locksmith, the middle-aged prostitute or the fishmonger's wife, a family of weavers and a family of orphans.

In contrast to the approach taken by Keith Wrightson, who was attracted to write about the 1636 plague in Newcastle-upon-Tyne by the documents penned by one person,[5] many sources have been used in the research for this book. This is one of the advantages of working in Cambridge, as sources relevant to the 1665 plague can be found in the Cambridgeshire Archives, the Cambridgeshire Collection, Cambridge University Library and college archives. Another advantage is that the layout of the streets in central Cambridge is the same as it was in 1665, and many of the houses where plague victims lived still exist.

CHAPTER 1

The Black Horse of the Apocalypse
and its Pale Rider

O N 25 July 1665 five-year-old John Morley of Holy Trinity parish in Cambridge died. On his chest were found black spots, tokens of the plague. His little brother, who had sat on a stool round-eyed and fearful watching him, also had spots on his face: he was swept from his mother's arms by men dressed in white robes and taken away. He died in the pest house on 5 August 1665, and the distraught parents were shut up in their house with a red cross painted on the door and the words 'Lord Have Mercy on Us' written below it. In Cambridge, the nightmare had begun.[1]

Although the inhabitants of Cambridge might have basked in the summer sun of 1665, at the back of their minds was the unspoken fear of plague. A pestilence that spread through a community like wildfire as the Black Horse of the Apocalypse with its pale rider picked off its victims. People died from painful tumours in the armpit and groin, from deadly fevers and blood poisoning. There was no known cure, and many saw the pestilence as heralding the end of the world as towns and villages were deserted and the dead lay in the streets with no one left to bury them.

The Black Death as it later became known was first seen in England in July 1348, when a ship carrying infected sailors docked at Melcombe Regis in Dorset. By April 1349 the plague was in Cambridge.[2] But by 1350 plague deaths ceased, and the country breathed a collective sigh of relief. The crisis was over and life could get back to normal, or as normal as it could be when houses stood empty, fields lay untilled, there were gaps in the tavern, and familiar faces missing from the pumps where women met to draw water and do their washing.

In Cambridge work started on three new colleges to train men for the priesthood and replace those who had died in the plague. Bishop Bateman of Norwich founded Trinity Hall and completed Gonville Hall, and in 1352 Corpus Christi College was founded by the town's gilds and their patron John of Gaunt, Duke of Lancaster.[3] For a time there was full employment in the town, more scholars arrived at the university, there was enough food for everyone, and widows and widowers, agreeing that it was better to share life, remarried. This time of reconstruction was not to last, however, and the plague returned to the town in 1361. It was to reappear in every century of the millennium. In 1447 Henry VI cancelled a visit to Cambridge to lay the foundation stone of King's College because 'of the air of pestilence which has long reigned in our said university', and in 1511 the humanist scholar Erasmus left London because of the plague and was trapped in Cambridge until 1513 'in the midst of pestilence and hemmed in by robbers'.[4]

When plague appeared in the town, the university suspended lectures and sent the students away. Stourbridge Fair, held on the outskirts of Cambridge, was cancelled by royal proclamation, all entertainment was banned and the social and economic life of the town was severely disrupted. In the seventeenth century if rumours of plague in London reached Cambridge, the town tried to isolate itself and forbade all contact with the capital. On 9 July 1625 Mr Mead of Christ's College, Cambridge wrote to Sir Martin Stuteville in London, 'It grows very dangerous on both sides to continue an intercourse by letter, not knowing what hands they pass through. Our Hobson and others have been forbidden to go to London.' He added, 'Blessed be to God, we are yet well at Cambridge.' He was too optimistic; on 28 August 1625 the mayor's feast was cancelled because of the plague, and on 20 October all sermons and public assemblies were banned.[5]

The Hobson mentioned in the letter was Thomas Hobson, the university carrier, livery stable keeper, town benefactor and one of seventeenth-century Cambridge's more colourful characters. This is the Hobson of 'Hobson's Choice', taken from his practice of hiring out his horses in strict rotation and not allowing his customers to choose, regardless of whether the next horse on the rota was an elderly nag or a spirited young blood too frisky for the customer to control.

Thomas Hobson took over the carrier's business in 1568 and soon proved to be an adept businessman, expanding the business so that a fleet of his carts carried goods, passengers, letters and packages as well as the university's mail and parcels between Cambridge and London. As his business grew so did his wealth, and he began to invest in property in Cambridge and in the surrounding countryside, including Anglesey Abbey, and land in Cottenham and Waterbeach. In 1628 he conveyed land in St Andrew's Street in Cambridge to the town and the university, and provided money to build and equip a workhouse for poor women, which became known as the Spinning House. He also paid for a conduit into the Market Place into which pure spring water flowed from Trumpington Nine Wells.

This was part of a scheme jointly designed by the town and the university to have a flow of fresh water through the streets to cleanse the town and, it was hoped, prevent further outbreaks of disease. (The flow of water can still be seen in Trumpington Street, but the conduit has been moved to the corner of Trumpington Street and Lensfield Road.)

Hobson died during the plague outbreak, but not of the plague. The poet John Milton who was studying at Christ's College at the time thought it was because Hobson could not stand the inaction when forbidden to travel to London, and dedicated a poem to him, 'On the University Carrier Who Sickened in the Time of His Vacancy, being Forbid to go to London, by Reason of the Plague.'[6]

Prior to 1665 the worst outbreak of plague Cambridge had experienced occurred in 1630 and 1631. This was within living memory of many people living in Cambridge in 1665, and others had been told about it by their parents or grandparents. Alderman Samuel Newton of Cambridge, who was to keep a diary from 1662 to 1717, was aged five during the 1630 outbreak and in his late teens during the plagues of 1642 and 1646 so he could remember what it was like to live in a town where pestilence stalked the streets. It was not surprising that, having endured 1665, when plague returned to the town in 1666 he upped sticks and moved his family to Waterbeach in the countryside.[7]

Others heard of it from their parents or grandparents. They were told how people starved because the country folk were too frightened to bring their produce into town, and how daily hundreds of people trooped out of the town to the fields to find grain. They were told how the university's vice-chancellor Dr Butts tried to help the infected sick and the poor, giving them money and employing a German physician to minister to the sick in the pest house, and provided bedding and firing from his own purse. They were told how by May 1630 at least 222 people had died of the plague, and there were nearly 3,000 people on poor relief.[8]

Children were told by their grandparents how, when all hope was lost, a letter was read out in all the parish churches in England asking for a collection to be made for the destitute poor of Cambridge, and money poured in from cities, towns and villages. It came from communities stricken with the plague themselves – £20 from Leicester, £100 from the county of Essex, £57 from St Neots; even tiny villages sent as much as they could afford, and eventually £2,739 7s. 4d was collected (over £200,000 in today's money). The corporation began to disburse this in March 1631 and the crisis was over.[9]

The town had survived one of its worst periods, and it was to survive further outbreaks of the plague in 1637 and 1638, and again in 1642 and 1646 when Cambridge was a garrison town during the Civil War. Then the plague appeared to cease, but by the 1660s 'there was a notion among the common people that the plague visited every 20 years and must return'.[10] Henry More, a tutor at Christ's College, Cambridge wrote to Lady Conway on 4 January 1663:

> ... and I am afraid a great mortality is coming upon these Nations. The weather here is as if it were April or May for warmth. Primroses and violets have been a-bloom a good while; the birds sing as in Spring in the orchard. I believe we shall have an ill after-reckoning of all this mirth ... There have been many fiery Meteors seen, several rivers and wells dry'd which show that there have been considerable changes in the Entrails of the Earth. I wish these things be not forerunners of some greater Mortality ...[11]

Astrologers predicted the plague's reappearance because of the conjunction of Saturn and Jupiter in Sagittarius on 9 October 1664 and between Mars and Saturn on 12 November.[12] Astrological predictions were confirmed on 12 November 1664 by the appearance of a harbinger of doom, a comet.

Samuel Newton saw the comet in Cambridge on 17 December 1664:

> The same day in the morning from about 2 of the clock to 5 in the morning was seen in the air a Comet, which several days latterly has also been seen: the star itself was very little or not at all bigger than an ordinary star, it had a ray which appeared in the judgement of some to be 20 yards in length, to others the length of a pike, to others the length of King's College Chapel, it appeared south east wards.

He saw the comet again on 3 April 1665 at three in the morning, as he was rising early to go to Hog's Hill.[13] Some thought that a visitation from the plague was a 'stroke of God's wrath for the sins of Mankind', and a broom to sweep the kingdom clean.[14] It was no accident that some of the symptoms of the plague resembled those of venereal disease, the mark of a dissolute life and corrupt society where sexual excess and depravity were common. Others thought that a dose of the clap could be a preventive against the plague and went out of their way to catch it.[15]

The most popular theory on the cause of the plague was miasma, 'the earth belching forth venomous vapours' – vapours caused by filth, overcrowding, dunghills, excrement, stinking standing water, putrefying churchyards all polluting the air. The vapours could lie dormant in the soil during cold weather and resurface when it became warmer.[16] This was borne out by the patterns of plague deaths which decreased in the winter, only to occur in greater numbers in the summer.

The idea that bad air could cause disease persisted into the nineteenth century, but we now know that plague was caused by a bacillus, *Yersinia pestis*, identified by Dr Alexandre Yersin in 1894.

Helped by the new science of bacteriology he found that the bacillus that caused plague was primarily a disease of rats. Four years later P. Simond recognised that the disease spread to humans through the bite of a rat flea. He found that once the rat host died, the infected flea left to find another warm body to feed on, but as it could not ingest any blood, when it bit the human it injected the lethal bacillus under the skin. Plague was transmitted from flea bites rather than from human to human.[17] However, a secondary infection of the lungs, or pneumonic plague could be spread from human to human by droplets.[18] This was the type of plague referred to in the nursery rhyme 'Ring a ring o' roses'. The 1665–66 outbreak was almost certainly bubonic plague. William Boghurst records from his observations of plague victims that there was little of the sneezing that there had been in other countries and other times.[19]

There was no known cure for the scourge, but the medical profession had many preventive measures that could be used. That august body, the College of Physicians suggested that prevention of the plague started with prayer and repentance, and, if it became necessary to go out into the streets, tobacco, rue or angelica should be chewed and clothes should be perfumed with juniper or cedar wood. Pomanders should be hung around the neck. The college helpfully gave two recipes, one for the poor and one for the rich. The pomander for the poor was made of rue, zedoary (turmeric), myrrh, 2 grains of camphor and 2 grains of laudanum put into a cloth bundle. The richer sort's pomander included citron pills, angelica seeds, zedoary, rose leaves, aloes, 5 grains of laudanum, and 5 drachms of gum dissolved in rose-water and enclosed in an ivory box to be hung on a golden chain.[20] Oranges studded with cloves tended to be a more temporary solution.

The college also published a selection of diets that could be used as a preventive. These ranged from fasting to eating a great deal of garlic cooked in butter with bread and sage or summer sorrel. London or Venetian treacle was considered especially beneficial. This was not treacle as we know it, but a compound of seventy-five ingredients, each added with great ceremony and the result taken as a pill.[21]

Non-medical practitioners had their own recipes. Hannah Glasse prescribed plague water. This was an infusion of rue, sage, mint, rosemary, wormwood and lavender in a gallon of wine, which was put into a pot and left to warm in ashes for four or five days, then strained and bottled with camphor. It could be taken by mouth, rubbed on the loins or the temple, or sniffed up. A similar recipe appears in the recipe book of the Barnadistons, a family of apothecaries in Bury St Edmunds. They boiled rue and sugar in muscardine wine and added nutmeg, pepper, treacle and angelica water. Half a spoonful was to be taken in the morning and half in the evening, and then trust in God.[22]

When plague was identified the Privy Council swung into action and issued a series of orders to county sheriffs and town councils. The first set of directives was concerned with stopping the infection from spreading, banning all public meetings and cancelling fairs, including Cambridge's Stourbridge Fair. The next order stated that all streets and alleys were to be thoroughly cleansed and fires strewn with sweet herbs were to burn on street corners. No dogs, cats or tame pigeons were allowed out on the streets, and some authorities went so far as to kill all dogs, cats and pigeons in their town. Infected households were to be closed up or the inhabitants sent to a pest house. Wardens were to be appointed to watch infected houses and supply necessities, and searchers were to be appointed to identify plague victims. Lastly, there were to be monthly fasts, public prayers every Wednesday and Friday, and collections made in churches for the infected poor, 'by which means God may be inclined to remove his severe hand from amongst you and us'.[23]

Towns took these orders seriously and isolated the infected poor in pest houses, which at first were hastily erected sheds where the dead and the dying were close neighbours, but later were purpose-built structures. There were four pest houses in Cambridge: at Ball's Folly/Gonville Place, Midsummer Common, Jesus Green, and the largest at Coldham Common on the eastern outskirts of the town. The pest houses were often left to decay on the site, but in April 1658 the university and town agreed that in case the town should be visited by sickness again they would be prepared by building timber cabins on commons and waste places in the town at their joint expense. These would follow the pattern of the sheds built on Coldham Common, consisting of two timber frames with six lodging rooms, and in every room a brick chimney and an iron bar to hang pots from. The external walls were to be of brick, two and a half yards high, well covered with tiles and sealed with hair mortar and the rooms to be paved with brick. Each room was to have a door with a lock and windows with wooden shutters. There was to be separate accommodation for overseers and watchers. The cost of building these came to £189 1s. 9½d. Despite this building programme, on 22 November 1663 the corporation noted that many of the pest houses were in bad condition and would deteriorate further unless they were properly repaired.[24] Few survived the move to a pest house and contemporaries thought it a 'A Slaughter house for Mankind'.[25]

This is what the inhabitants of Cambridge had to look forward to in 1665: a disease without any known cure which could spread like wildfire through the town, and a painful death, either shut up in their own houses with the dead and dying, or locked in a pest house.

CHAPTER 2

FINE BUILDINGS AND BAD SMELLS

IN SEPTEMBER 1654 the diarist and gardener John Evelyn rode into Cambridge from Huntingdon. He came along the old Roman road, through Fenstanton, across the Fens with the church towers of Lolworth and Fen Drayton in the distance, through the fields of Girton and across the West Fields of Cambridge with their stubble after the harvest and before the winter ploughing. He rode past the Civil War bastions defending Cambridge Castle, and passed the castle mound. Here an unpleasant smell assailed him from one of the common dunghills situated in a valley behind the castle.[1] On his left was the parish church of St Giles, and on his right St Peter's parish with its fish ponds and willows.[2] He rode past Magdalene College and across the Great Bridge over the Cam, which gives the town its name. The ducking stool for scolds hung from this bridge, suspended over the river by a pulley on a beam; the back of the stool, which faced the road, was engraved and painted with devils laying hold of scolds.[3]

Visitors from London, such as Samuel Pepys, entered the town through flat open fenland grazed by cattle and sheep, and like

St Peter's parish heavily fringed with willows. Willows were an important cash crop in Cambridge, and a map of 1688 by David Loggan shows every watercourse and every road shaded by them, with at least 200 stands of these trees on Coe Fen and St Thomas Leys; Celia Fiennes who visited the town in 1685 described it as 'garnished with willows'.[4] Visitors from east came into Cambridge from the Gog Magog Hills, the highest point overlooking the town. On a clear day King's College Chapel and Ely Cathedral could be seen from the hills, but when Daniel Defoe rode to Cambridge 'the Isle of Ely look'd as if wrapp'd in Blankets, and nothing to be seen . . .'[5]

Each entrance to the town was marked by a common dunghill. As well as at the castle others stood at the country end of Jesus Lane, at Spital End on the Trumpington road, and in the west close to Newnham Mill and the ancient house known as The Hermitage.[6] Household waste, manure, rotting vegetation and dead dogs and cats were deposited on the dunghills, and the stench from these mingled with the smell of blood from Fair Lane and Slaughter House Lane, where the butchers went about their business. Even more pungent and obvious was the odour from Robert Atkinson's Scalding House, where hair and fibres were scalded off animals' bodies.[7]

It was not the smell of the town that visitors commented on, but the air. John Evelyn described it as 'thick, infested by the fens', and William Schellink a Dutchman travelling in England between 1661 and 1663 wrote, 'There is nothing lacking but better air, which because of the vapours from bog lands, is somewhat unhealthy, especially in summer when it is heavy and murky.'[8] The bad air was caused by fen fogs and coal smoke which, due to the low-lying position of Cambridge, combined to form evil-smelling smog, or miasma; and of course as miasma was thought to be one of the main causes of the plague, Cambridge was seen as an especially unhealthy place and one which was prone to pestilence.

Coal fires and the industrial hearths in the little workshops behind the houses in the town created a distinctive urban smell. Christopher Bumstead's brazier's workshop behind his house in Holy Sepulchre parish had a hearth permanently lit, and the sound of him beating metal echoed round the streets. William Key, a locksmith, had a small workshop and hearth in All Saints parish, and numerous farriers and smiths in the town added to the smells and sounds of the streets. In Newmarket Road, Richard Sanders, a blacksmith, rented the Leper Chapel to use as his forge, conveniently placed to catch travellers into town or visiting Stourbridge Fair.[9]

Coal was the preferred fuel in Cambridge. There was little timber available for logs and firewood in the area, and although peat could be dug from the Fens, this was used in conjunction with coal. Coal was distributed to the poor as fuel, and was used as a commodity with which to speculate.[10] A Bill in Chancery shows that coal for Cambridge was purchased in King's Lynn and delivered by water to the Common Hythe in St Clement's parish, and sold from there.[11]

King's Lynn was linked to Cambridge by the Rivers Cam and Ouse, and the town was also a hub on the road from the north and the Midlands via Huntingdon (now the A1M and A14) and through to East Anglia and the port of Harwich. Travellers who rode into Cambridge were not impressed with the roads. William Schellink arrived in a heavy rainstorm and took lodgings at the Lion, which stood opposite St John's College. On his way to the town from London he encountered throngs of coaches and people leaving Stourbridge Fair to return to the city, and complained that this made the road wet and muddy and almost impossible to traverse.[12]

It took two days to reach Cambridge from London on horse-back,[13] but in 1653 the first coach left Cambridge for London. It departed from the Devil's Tavern (now the site of Senate House) and took twelve hours to complete the journey. It was so successful that it was joined by a second coach in 1655. Known as 'The Fly', this left the Swan in Gray's Inn Road, Holborn for the Rose in Cambridge every Monday, Wednesday and Friday, and returned from the Rose every Tuesday, Thursday and Saturday. The fare was 10s. single, and it would carry letters and packets for customers.[14] Numerous carriers also plied between Cambridge and London, and their heavy wagons were partly responsible for the poor state of the roads. Many carriers were licensed letter-carriers for the university; in the early 1660s they included Roger Greene, Roger Hurst of St Edward's parish, and Henry Glenton of Great St Mary's parish, but the most important was William Waterson who ran his business from a bay at the east end of a building called the Purgold on Pease Hill. Their licences included prices for delivering letters: 2d for letters weighing 1 ounce, and 3d for letters above this weight.[15]

Heavy goods came by river and hythes (wharfs) clustered along its banks, each catering for a different commodity – Corn Hythe, Flax Hythe, Garlic Hythe, Salt Hythe and, for general purposes, Dame Nichol's Hythe and the Common Hythe. Narrow lanes led from the hythes to the High Street and Market Place, and sixteenth- and seventeenth-century maps show that these often crossed college grounds. The rumble of handcarts as the porters brought goods up from the river added to the sound of horses' hooves on paved and cobbled streets and the iron-shod wheels of carts and coaches leaving the Rose and the Devil's Tavern; all formed part of the strident noise of a seventeenth-century town.

Two major bridges spanned the river, the Great Bridge on the road to Huntingdon and the Little Bridge by Queens' College on the road to Newnham, while colleges had private bridges over the river, and a public pedestrian bridge led to Garrett Hostel Green, between Trinity College and Trinity Hall.[16] The river was more than a communication artery; people washed themselves and their clothes in it, having been forbidden by the corporation to wash in the brooks or the town streets 'but only in the river'.[17] Townspeople and scholars fished in it (tiny fishermen are shown on a sixteenth-century map), wildfowl were shot on its banks, and people boated on it for pleasure. Scholars and townsmen swam in it – one portion of the town fen by the river was known as the 'swimming croft' – and sewage was discharged into it, which added to the town's pungency in summer.[18]

A 15-foot-wide man-made watercourse known as the King's Ditch encircled the town. This left the river at Mill Lane, crossed Pembroke Street and St Andrew's Street, then ran down Hobson Street before it was crossed by a chain bridge in Walls Lane, went across the back of Sidney Sussex College, under Jesus Lane in a culvert, and down Park Street to rejoin the river opposite Magdalene College.[19] The ditch was dug in 1274, and its purpose is unknown. It could have been defensive, or it could have been intended as part of a drainage system, but it was a body of stagnant water which posed a permanent health hazard, especially as the town had no obligation to clean it, and refuse, muck, dead animals and night soil were thrown into it, so it posed a breeding ground for insects and vermin, and one of the most unpleasant sights in the town.

A succession of maps from 1574 to 1688 shows that the layout of Cambridge had changed little during that time, and the plan of the central area was similar to that which exists today: Bridge Street which runs from the Great Bridge to St Andrew's Street with a branch to Jesus Lane, the High Street, now known as Trinity Street and King's Parade, and Milne Street which in the seventeenth century led from the mills at the south end of the town opposite Queens' College, across the King's College and Trinity College grounds, of which a fossilised section can be seen between the Old Schools and Clare College and at the back of Gonville and Caius College.[20]

The Market Place was the commercial hub of the town. In the seventeenth century it was rectangular in shape, with a row of permanent shops and stalls in the north-east, and the Market Cross in the south at the junction of Pease Hill and Market Hill. The market cross was raised on a flight of stone steps, and at one time had a wooden roof over it, but by 1660 only the steps and the shaft remained, and in 1664 it had to be rebuilt.[21] When Samuel Newton was town treasurer in 1664 on 1 October he had to collect 1d from every butcher's and fish stall in the market. He collected 9s. 3d,[22] which works out as 111 stalls in total.

Hobson's Conduit stood at the centre of the market. On the west side was Great St Mary's church, with shops and houses abutting its west end. These included Leonard Green's printer's shop, and Thomas Buck the university printer.[23] The town hall was on the south side of the market with the Tolbooth and gaol beside it. The town hall had an open arcade with stalls beneath it, and a kitchen on the first floor, reached by an open staircase.[24] The corn market was on the north side of the Market Place and Slaughter Lane, Butchers' Row and the beast market were on the south-west. Here was the smell of death, the moaning of terrified animals, and the sight of blood and offal in the streets' drains. Other sounds in this area were the baying for blood from the Bull Ring on Pease Hill, and that of the cockfights held in surrounding inns.

Oats and fish were sold on Pease Hill, and in Butter Row. Temporary stalls were set up in the centre of the market, and women from the countryside sold butter and eggs from the steps of the market cross. Every morning the market was proclaimed open by the crier with his handbell, accompanied by the mayor's sergeant of the mace and the university proctors. The proclamation ordered 'All persons that dwell in the town or shall repair to it to keep the King's Peace, and not make affray or outcry, or wear any weapons', and exhorted 'all bakers to bake good bread, all ale-sellers and vintners to sell good measure, all butchers to sell good and wholesome flesh, and all chandlers to make good candles without mixing kitchen stuff in the tallow, and to sell at a rate set by the university'.[25]

Once the market was open there were cries from market traders, and street sellers hawking their pies and pasties from trays on their heads, there were pleas from beggars for alms, there was the sound of feet: old men shuffling with sticks, apprentices with iron-shod shoes running on errands, or bouncing pigs' bladders looking for a game of football. There was the sound of the treble voices of little boys playing with clay marbles in the gutter or rolling wooden hoops down the streets, or made by little girls with their dolls and skipping ropes. There were ladies of stately gait with pet dogs, and the shouts of men with hunting dogs going into the surrounding fields to shoot game, punctuating the sounds of the town with gunshot.

The lanes branching off the Market Place carried the names of the trades originally practised there; Shoemakers' Row, for example, or Shearers Lane. Upmarket shops stood on Market Hill, Richard and John Clay's upholsterer's shop next door to James Sadler's draper's emporium, and close to John Pepys's confectionary, while Southhouse Robinson a tobacco-pipe maker lived in Great Fair Yard, next door to John Ilger an alderman, and Edward Miller's Red Lyon Inn.[26]

Most essential commodities and some luxuries could be purchased in the vicinity: gloves at John Bishop's shop across the river close to Newnham Mill, and shoes from one of the seven shoemakers in town. Clothes could be made to measure, meat and bread could be acquired, as could household necessities such as nails made by Henry Clerk in his workshop in Castle End. You could get your hair cut by William Jones a barber with premises in Harleston Lane in St Clement's parish, buy a fish from Peter Lightfoot, have your windows mended by the Woodward family, and if you were ill there were two physicians, Dr Robert Eade and Dr Edward Stoyle, and at least three apothecaries: Peter Dent, Artemus Hinde and William Frisby.[27]

The first thing a visitor to seventeenth-century Cambridge might have noticed was the contrast between the stone-built colleges and churches and the timber-framed houses with wattle and daub walls and thatched or tiled roofs, often in bad repair and needing fresh plaster and a lick of paint. The fire hazard in a town like this was enormous, so every parish and college had to keep fire-fighting equipment and take an annual inventory of it. The equipment included ladders, buckets, fire hooks for dragging down thatched roofs, and some parishes had an engine for pumping water. These precautions paid off and there was no major conflagration in the town during the last half of the seventeenth century.

The larger houses were usually of three storeys with attics and jetties overhanging the streets; more modest houses had a ground floor and an attic used for sleeping and storage. Maps from the late sixteenth century show the larger houses set within their own grounds, but by 1688 David Loggan's map shows solid blocks of housing, gardens and yards in-filled with cottages huddled together.

There was little privacy in this overcrowded situation, and the quarrels and uproar of antisocial neighbours filtered through thin wattle and daub walls. Revellers coming home at night disturbed the sleep of decent citizens, and the cries of women in labour could be heard by neighbours and passers-by as all windows and doors were thrown open as sympathetic magic to ease labour pains. The groans of the dying echoed through the streets, and when plague came it was announced by the slamming of the house door and the hammering of boards across it to stop anyone inside escaping, and followed all too soon by the rumble of the parish bier.

Some of the largest buildings in Cambridge were the inns. Many of these were on the approach roads, the Black Bull and Cardinal's Cap in Trumpington Street on the road in from London, while the Swan and the White Horse (now the Folk Museum) were on the road from Huntingdon. Across the Great Bridge, Bridge Street was lined with inns and taverns, the Blackamoor Head, the Mitre, the Salutation, the Bull, and the Peacock and the Crow where the Griggs brothers were landlords. Travellers coming by water or porters unloading goods on the common wharf could get a drink and a room for the night at the Old Ship, the Sun, the Anchor or the Magpie, while for locals there was the Nine Pins in Thompson's Lane. Roger Thompson's brewery was situated in St Clement's parish, and the Swan across the river also had its own brewery; in the same vicinity was St John's College brewery.[28] The distinctive yeasty smell of brewing permeated the town, as did the unpleasant odour as chandlers rendered down fat to make candles.

Close to the Market Place was the Eagle and Child in Bene't Street (now the Eagle) next door to the Cross Keys, and nearby were the Three Feathers, another Mitre whose landlord was Alderman Owen Mayfield, and the very uninviting Dunghill. Clustered round the market and Petty Cury were the Falcon, the Red Lion and the Wrestlers owned by William Crane a scrivener. There was the Angel in Market Passage, the Raven in Shoemakers' Row, and the Rose (on the site of what is now Rose Crescent). The Bird Bolt Inn whose landlady was Elizabeth Gill was close to Emmanuel College, the Blue Bell stood in Walls Lane (now King Street) and across Barnwell Fields was the Brazen George.[29]

Places designated as inns sold food and drink and provided lodgings. The food included spit roasts, savoury pies and pasties, and sugar cakes which were especially popular in Cambridge. Some inns put on entertainment for their guests, as recorded by Samuel Pepys when he was staying at the Rose in 1667. 'The town music did also come and play, but Lord! What a sad music they made.'[30] Cambridge was a town of music, from the town and university waits performing in the streets to the pipes and fiddles celebrating May Day and the coming of summer.

Appetising smells came from the cook shops in Petty Cury, of roasting meats, ripe cheeses, and in winter of mulled ale combined with the sound of fat dripping onto hot coals to attract the hungry passer-by. A French visitor to England in the late seventeenth century left a description of a cook shop where four spits turned day and night, each with five or six pieces of butcher's meat on it – beef, mutton, pork, veal or lamb. The customers chose the cut they wanted, fat or lean, rare or well done, and it was served with salt, mustard, a bread roll and beer. Misson described this as a feast,[31] and the cook shop seems to be the early forerunner of the kebab shop or hamburger joint.

The town was divided into four wards, Market Ward, High Ward which extended from St John's College to Trumpington Street, Bridge Ward which covered the area from the north end of Jesus Lane and crossed the river to the castle, and Preacher's Ward which went from the south side of Jesus Lane to St Andrew's Street. Within the wards were fourteen separate parishes and parish churches. The most important of these, Great St Mary's, which stood on the west side of the Market Place and was shared by the university and the corporation, was the scene of many bitter squabbles over precedence. Also close to the market was the parish of St Edward, King and Martyr, and a little further south St Bene't's parish. St Botolph and Little St Mary's parishes were by the old Trumpington Gate, and St Michael's was on the High Street, as was All Saints parish in the seventeenth century (the parish church was moved to Jesus Lane in the nineteenth century). Holy Trinity parish covered Shoemakers' Row and the surrounding streets, and Bridge Ward was divided into

Holy Sepulchre or the Round Church parish, St Clement and, across the river, St Peter and St Giles parishes.

Each of these churches had its own graveyard. It was in the parish church that the vital events in the parishioners' lives took place and were recorded in the parish registers. Parishioners were married in the parish church, baptised their children there, and were laid to rest in its churchyard. Much of parish life revolved around this church, and the minister and churchwardens would have been familiar figures to everyone, and because the Act for the Better Relief of the Poor of 1662 made poor relief available only to those legally settled in the parish, the churchwardens as overseers of the poor would have known who their parishioners were, and who was a stranger or incomer.

The sound of church bells marked the passing seasons. All bells, town and university's, rang out to mark the anniversary of the Gunpowder Plot on 5 November, to celebrate the birthday of the monarch, and to mark the Restoration of Charles II, and his coronation day. Individual parishes tolled the passing bell to announce the death of a parishioner; a stroke for every year of life plus ten for a male, and one for each year of life for a female. Peals rang out to summon parishioners to church on a Sunday, and to announce marriages and important national events; the church bells were interspersed with the town crier's handbell as he went around the town informing the inhabitants about what was happening in the town, and when they should put a light outside their doors to illuminate dark streets. The town's bells were echoed by the village bells of St Andrew the Less in Barnwell across open fields from the town, and Chesterton church north of the river.

The streets were full of the smell of people; of sweaty unwashed bodies and clothes. Washing the person and clothes was difficult in the seventeenth century and although Cambridge allowed the washing of clothes in the river, there was much to deter people from doing this, not least the state of the river, while clothes and bedding made of wool and linen were difficult to wash and keep clean. Soap was made from the fat left over by the tallow chandlers and not suitable for use on the skin, and only the very wealthy could afford soft soap. John Evelyn recorded washing his hair once a year, and Samuel Pepys preferred a rub down to a wet wash.[32] Bad breath would have been a universal problem. Some people chewed sweet herbs to disguise this, or used a mouthwash of spearmint or cloves, and some tried to clean their teeth with salt, soot or a bunch of twigs. A diet based on bread, beer, cheese and meat led to a great deal of flatulence, but much of this was masked by the smell of tobacco, and smoking was extremely popular in seventeenth-century Cambridge, and an essential part of civic life.[33] Of course, the regular intake of tobacco caused much coughing and spitting, about which there were no corporation orders.

The sights that drew the crowd together could be a corporation procession, the men in scarlet gowns and preceded by the town's mace-bearer, or the scold dipped on the ducking stool from the Great Bridge, the forger in the pillory, or fornicators in the stocks. Here was an opportunity to let off steam and pelt the miscreants with rotten fruit, vegetables, stones and other rubbish. Accidents, too, drew a crowd. If a cart turned over a crowd soon gathered to give advice, or if a horse slipped on the greasy cobbles, and if a pie man stumbled and spilled his load, there was a golden opportunity for free food.

Scurrying through the streets on their way to lectures or the nearest tavern were the members of the university, and it was the colleges that helped to attract visitors to Cambridge. Not only to talk to men of learning, but to gasp at the magnificence of King's College Chapel, or to compare Cambridge unfavourably with Oxford. John Evelyn thought St Catharine's College a 'mean structure' and Jesus College in a 'melancholy state', while Celia Fiennes judged Trinity College to be fine 'but not as fine as Christ Church, Oxford'.[34]

There were sixteen colleges in seventeenth-century Cambridge, each within its own enclosed space which included gardens, pleasant groves, and bowling greens and tennis courts for recreation. Today colleges front the street, but in the seventeenth century, when they were much smaller, town houses stood between the colleges and the street, so, for example, the green in front of King's College was filled with cottages.

In the 1660s when Isaac Newton studied in Cambridge there were three essential units in the college: the college chapel, library and hall,[35] set within cloisters. Open staircases led to the upper storeys where fellows and students lived. During the hard winters of the 1660s college rooms, open cloisters and corridors would have been intensely cold. The wind cut across Cambridge and its colleges, bringing ice, frost and snow, and the open staircases became death traps. The Hearth Tax returns show that there were 215 hearths in Trinity College.[36] While he was a student at Trinity, Isaac Newton spent 11s. on six and a half sacks of coal and turf in 1667, and it cost St John's College £120 a year to heat the public rooms in the college with coal, sedge and turf. Candles were another expense for the college and individual students, and a constant bone of contention with the town, as the university fixed the price of candles; Isaac Newton paid 6d a pound for his candles, and 1s. 11d for a candlestick.[37]

One feature a visitor from today might notice in a seventeenth-century college was the all-pervading smell of horse. Colleges had their own stable, grooms and blacksmiths. Thomas Ingery was a groom in the Trinity College stables. He lived in a single room in college where he slept and cooked on an open fire.[38]

The college year started with the Great Commencement in June, and then the scholars left for the Long Vacation, returning in time for Stourbridge Fair. The year was punctuated by college feasts and entertainments, and the college hall, with a dais at one end, could quickly be converted into a theatre with a stage on which plays could be performed. Although Isaac Newton tended to ignore it, attendance at the college chapel or another place of worship was almost compulsory. Especial attention was paid to the Thanksgiving service on 5 November which was followed by bonfires, and other anniversaries such as the monarch's birthday or coronation day. By the mid-seventeenth century these had taken over from the old calendar of saints' days, although college feasts might coincide with the appropriate saint's day.

The colleges were part of the university and the university had privileges, granted to it by successive monarchs, which gave it substantial power over the town that each new mayor had to swear to uphold. This included control over all official weights and measures, its own court where women apprehended by the proctors on suspicion of prostitution could be tried, the right to license or prohibit all actors, wrestlers, bear-baiters and jesters in the town or for five miles around. It could set the price of commodities such as candles and ban any tradesmen who allowed students to run up unacceptable debts, from trading with the university or with colleges.[39] These privileges gave rise to tension between the town and the university, which could lead to riots, as it did in 1662 when a Royal Commission arrived to purge the members of the town's corporation who had supported Parliament in the Civil War. The commission appointed a new mayor and corporation without an election, which usurped one of the town's most closely guarded privileges. The town blamed the university for this, riots followed and the university's vice-chancellor was mobbed by an angry crowd.[40] But the university and the town could work together in times of crisis, such as an outbreak of the plague, and town and gown were tied together by economic necessity. The university and the colleges provided employment, and the town provided them with people, goods and services. Town and gown lived in a symbiotic relationship.

Another reason that visitors flocked to the town was to attend Stourbridge Fair, and Cambridge's year was enlivened by four fairs. The first was Reach Fair, held in May. Although Reach was twelve miles from Cambridge the fair was the property of the town burgesses and was proclaimed open by the Mayor of Cambridge. The next fair in the Cambridge calendar was Midsummer Fair, also owned by the town. Held on Greencroft (now Midsummer Common), it was proclaimed open 'once against The Cock, and at the water fair beyond the soap barrels'.[41] It lasted a fortnight, and dealers came from the surrounding counties to sell knives, gloves, girdles and pots. Some came with contraband – unlicensed books. Joseph Townsend a haberdasher from Northampton not only brought haberdashery to the fair, but secreted in his pack 46 pamphlets, 126 horn books and four bound and stitched octavo books. Robert Duncalve of London, a stationer, came with six unlicensed bibles to sell, and William Squire of Bedford with two unlicensed bibles. They were each fined 2s. 6d (about £10 today).[42]

Midsummer Fair was followed at the beginning of August by Garlic Fair, which was owned by Jesus College and held for two days at the junction of Park Street and Jesus Lane at a site then known as Garlic Lane. These fairs were tasters for one of the largest and most important fairs in England, Stourbridge Fair.

Buyers and sellers from across Britain and the Continent came to this fair. The road from London was jammed with fair-goers, the town's population was swollen by thousands, and it was the biggest social and economic event in the town's calendar. Inns and taverns were full, tradesmen set up home in their booths at the fair, and those unable to find accommodation slept in barns, stables and haystacks. The booths were owned by the burgesses and aldermen of the town.

When Samuel Newton was made a burgess in 1661 he was allocated five booths at the fair, which he could lease out for a good rent;[43] in his will he left his booths to his son, and to the Mayor and Corporation of Cambridge.[44]

Policing the fair was the responsibility of both university and town, and the fair was proclaimed open by the mayor and aldermen in scarlet on horseback. The fair stood on a permanent site bounded by the river on one side and Newmarket Road on the other, and was laid out in permanent streets with the land in between sown with arable crops during the winter.[45] The streets were wide enough for the sellers to bring in their carts to unload and turn round, and each street or row had its own speciality. Garlic Row was for milliners, toys, cabinetmakers and perfumers. Linen drapers, silk men, ironmongers and clothiers from the West Riding of Yorkshire clustered in the Duddery. Hops from Kent were sold at the fair, as were Manchester wares, blankets and rugs from Kidderminster, knives from Sheffield, brass ware from Birmingham, shoes from Northamptonshire, and stockings from Leicestershire and Yorkshire. Timber was for sale from barges on the river, and booths and tents held pop-up taverns, coffee houses, alehouses and cook shops. Butchers, higglers, cheese sellers and bakers flocked into the fair every morning to sell their wares, and the whole was interspersed with men and women selling ale from jugs and cans, puppet shows, comedians, rope-dancers, plays and other entertainments. A great deal of illegal gambling took place, and on the last day a horse fair was held, and horse and foot races.[46]

As a student, Isaac Newton purchased an English Euclid and other books at Stoubridge Fair, and in 1664 he also purchased a prism there to try out the experiments in Descartes' Book of Colours. He made a small hole in his window shutter, darkened his room, and stood the prism between the window and the wall.

He found that instead of a circle of light he saw an oblong with semicircular ends, and concluded that Descartes was wrong.[47]

Each commodity brought into the fair was inspected by four men, two appointed by the university and two by the town. They wore red coats and before taking up their duties were charged by the vice-chancellor of the university 'to be careful to observe whether any unlawful cards or bowls are played, any flesh dressed on a fasting day, or any quarrel or fight takes place'. They also had to make sure that butter and cheese were sold by tested weights and measures, and to keep a list of names of lewd and suspected persons. They were allowed 6d a day for wages and 6d for a night shift, 'but no supper'.[48]

Offenders selling false measures, rancid butter or bad fish were taken before the fair court and given summary justice of a fine. By far the most common offence was selling beer from jugs that had not been measured: 60 per cent of all the cases heard in the fair court between 1655 and 1667 were for this. The second most common crime was selling cheese the sellers had not made themselves. Other infringements included selling wine above the set price, selling rotten fish, musty tobacco, hops or mustard seed, poor-quality oysters, and unmeasured cloth. There were four instances of drinking alcohol on a Sunday (which the appraisers actually observed), four illegal lotteries, and a dancing mare without a licence.[49]

When the fair ended, an army of men moved in to take down and pack away the booths and clear the area ready for ploughing; the crops grown on the site were always plentiful owing to the nitrogen put into the soil by fair-goers and animals. The fair was over for another year.

The fair was a great event for the town, and people looked forward to it through the dark winter months, but it was a potential pool for contagion. When plague struck in London, Stourbridge Fair was one of the first events to be cancelled by royal proclamation, and in

Cambridge the sights and sounds of the town changed. Instead of music, church bells and processions there was the sound of houses being closed up, the sight and sound of carts taking the infected to the pest house, and the rumble of death carts collecting corpses. There was the smell of tobacco smoke as people smoked ferociously as protection against the plague. There was the sight of red crosses on houses, searchers dressed in white going through the streets carrying long wands of office. Public assemblies were banned, and people shunned their neighbours. The streets lost their vibrancy, and trade came to a standstill.

CHAPTER 3

TOWN AND GOWN

THE SOCIETY OF seventeenth-century Cambridge was pyramid shaped with a small number of wealthy gentlemen at the top, and a broad base of poor and the labourers existing on subsistence wages at the bottom. The Hearth Tax and the corporation and college lease books show about forty-five individuals at the top of the pyramid, who described themselves as gentlemen in the Hearth Tax, and are described as such in the leases, but the title had no legal force. It could signify those who could live on their means without working, but at least ten of those described as gentlemen in the 1660s were gainfully employed; they included two town clerks Edward Lawe and Samuel Spalding, Owen Mayfield a vintner and innkeeper, Christopher Rose alderman and innkeeper, Mr Finch keeper of the Dolphin, Henry Rix a brewer, Thomas Tifford a butcher, Bryan Kitchingman an attorney and Samuel Newton and Richard Pettit public notaries.[1]

Below the gentlemen in the town pyramid were the tradesmen and shopkeepers, such as shoemakers, bakers, chandlers, booksellers and

28

representatives of many other trades which made Cambridge an important service centre. They supported journeymen and apprentices learning the trade, but the town was really run by the labouring poor, some employed full-time such as Toby Watson of number 4 Jesus Lane,[2] others casual labourers picking up work where they could. Their living was precarious, and often they were forced to join the bottom layer of the pyramid and ask for parish poor relief, or beg for alms.

The station in life of the various people who thronged Cambridge's streets was instantly recognisable from the clothes they wore. This was the age of the full-bottomed wig, and those who could afford it and had sufficient status would wear one, and carry a sword. Public notaries hurrying about their business wore black gowns with white bands at the neck. Tradesmen too were distinguished by their clothes, a leather apron for a blacksmith for example, but it was more the evidence of hard labour clinging to their garments which gave their trade away, the soot of the chimney sweep, blackened clothes, face and hands of the coalman, the paint spatter of the painter, blood-stained clothes of the butcher, or the plaster-encrusted plasterer. The poor wore such second-hand clothes as they could acquire through charity and donations from the poor relief fund.

Our eyes and ears into the life of the town, its corporation's feasts and fairs, are those of Alderman Samuel Newton who kept a diary from 1662 to 1717. Through him we can attend corporation common day meetings, ride to Reach Fair, go fishing with town councillors and celebrate Christmas, and we can meet other members of the corporation and their rather put-upon wives.[3] Samuel Newton was born in Cambridge in 1625. His father was either a painter or a printer.[4] Where Samuel was educated is not known, but at some point he must have studied law as he is a public notary by 1660. In that year he purchased his freedom of the town of Cambridge and became a burgess with the assent of burgesses Roger Wilson and

Edward Potter, and paid 100s. for the privilege, and another 15s. 1d when he took the oath at the town hall in 1661.[5] As he had to buy his freedom it would appear he did not serve an apprenticeship in the town. It was expensive but worth the money because at the same time he was granted five booths at Stourbridge Fair.[6]

Samuel married Sarah Welbore in St Edward's parish church in January 1659; both of them were living in that parish at the time. Their first son John was born on 20 October 1659, and baptised a week later.[7] The Newtons lived in a house at the east end of St Edward's church, facing on to Pease Hill. This may be the house with a courtyard shown on a sixteenth-century map, and Samuel was to extend his grounds when he leased a piece of wasteland next to the churchyard. The map suggests that Samuel's house had three storeys, and the Hearth Tax shows it had nine hearths.[8] Living close to the town hall and the Market Place, Samuel was nicely placed at the centre of town life.

As a public notary Samuel attested to deeds and made certified copies to render them authentic; he was also registrar of Pembroke College and an auditor for Trinity College. His post as registrar demanded that he kept a clear and concise register of the college's records and drew up orders as required using the correct legal termi-nology. In order to do this he needed a clear head, a good hand, an expert knowledge of the law, and the ability to spot fake documents. His writing in the diary is, for the seventeenth century, easy to read, and although he probably employed clerks to do the day to day work, many documents would have been in his own hand. The office of public notary was one open to corruption, as for a bribe the notary could swear that a deed was authentic when it was not. There is no evidence that Samuel ever did this, but he became wealthy and obvi-ously had good credit, as when in 1664 he became town treasurer he had to put up a bond of £500 to show that he would fulfil his office honestly, and his will shows that he amassed property in Cambridge and outside.[9]

The Newtons' house had a narrow frontage facing the street, and broadened out towards the rear. The front door opened on to a hall on one side of which was Newton's office and on the other a parlour for entertaining visitors. Behind the parlour was a room where the household and guests could dine. This must have been a large room, as when he was mayor Newton entertained the two town treasurers, four bailiffs, the town recorder Roger Pepys, the twelve aldermen and twenty-four members of the common council.

Over the ground floor were chambers, and above them attics and storage. It is probable that a covered gallery ran the length of the first floor, as this was a popular feature in seventeenth-century Cambridge. The kitchen in the yard would have been linked to the main house by the buttery and pantry. This was the business end of the house where Mrs Newton reigned supreme. Here were spits for roasting meat, cooking utensils, fire tongs, pokers, pots, pans and a large wooden table for preparing food. Herbs hung from the ceiling, and a stone copper stood in the corner for heating water.

Mrs Newton managed the household with the help of one maid-servant hired by the year. One, Frances Preston married before her year was out, and was replaced by Anne Beecham until the end of the year.[10] Many anonymous young women must have passed through the Newtons' kitchen, and Mrs Newton must have had daily helps coming in to clean, boys to turn and watch the spits, men to cart away ashes, and a laundress to help with the annual wash.

Day began for Mrs Newton when the light filtered through the curtains of the chamber where she slept, and she had to be up early, especially on a day when Samuel was riding on civic duty and had to be out of the house and on horseback by eight o'clock. His clothes, a coat, waistcoat, knee breeches, knitted stockings and white falling bands at the neck, were laid out ready the night before, and his black or scarlet gown had to be brushed to remove dust or mud, and inspected for snags, and any gold tuffets or gold lace that needed mending.

Mrs Newton tried to keep up with fashions which filtered down from London, which in the 1660s for the evening meant a low-cut bodice and lace jabot attached by pins or buttons to a taffeta skirt; for daytime she wore an old-fashioned bodice and skirt with coloured woollen stockings kept up by garters. When she went out marketing she slipped on wooden pattens over her shoes, so that she was raised above the mire of the streets (these were the equivalent of wedge soles), and because she was a modest woman, the wife of a respected and respectable lawyer, unlike her upper-class neighbours who went outside bare-headed, she wore a tall crowned hat with a broad brim, and sometimes covered her hair with a linen coif.[11]

Breakfast in the Newton household on an ordinary day was bread, cold meats, cheese or fish washed down with ale or non-alcoholic small beer. On feast days and holidays such as New Year, breakfast could include oysters and wine.[12] Breakfast over, Samuel went into his office, and Sarah began the housework.

The house was kept clean by manual labour. Beds – feather and flock mattresses with feather bolsters – had to be made, the floors needed to be swept, the carpets brushed and once a week the mattresses had to be turned. Hannah Glasse, the author of *The Art of Cookery Made Plain and Easy*, advised throwing a little sand over a room before sweeping, as that would gather up flock and dirt, and save bedding, pictures and all other furniture from dust. Water had to be fetched. Rain barrels stood in the yard, or water could be carried from the common pump in Pump Lane by King's College, or from Hobson's Conduit in the Market Place. Water was a problem in seventeenth-century households: not for drinking, as this was unsafe, but for washing and cleaning. Washing up cooking utensils was an enormous problem. In the Newton household there would have been many pewter dishes and tankards which had to be scoured with sand or granite powder and then plunged into hot water, or silver that needed constant attention to stop it from tarnishing. Rebecca Price, the author of *The Compleat Cook* published in 1681, advised scouring pewter plates with a strong lye using a flannel cloth, and then rinsing them with water which contained whitening. Afterwards they would be set by a fire to dry, and then polished.[13]

The Newtons' maid did most of the heavy work, while Sarah had to consider what to cook for the main meal of the day, dinner at noon. The meal was usually meat roasted on the spit, a savoury pie with bread and cheese, and ale or wine. Vegetables were rarely served, perhaps a salad or a dish of globe artichokes. The pies and bread could have come from a baker or cook shop, as not all seventeenth-century houses had an oven, although it is likely that a large establishment such as the Newtons' had an oven in its yard and did its own baking. We know that Mrs Herring, the wife of the mayor Richard Herring, had an oven and baked her own cakes when the aldermen came to call.[14]

Mid-morning Mrs Newton went shopping. She purchased goods in the units of pounds (lb) and ounces (oz). An ounce was the equivalent of 28 grams, and there were 16 ounces, or 453 grams, to a pound. When she bought cloth for a new skirt or cloak, it was measured in feet and inches, each inch being 2.5 centimetres; a foot was 12 inches or 30.48 centimetres and a yard or three feet was 91.5 centimetres. She paid for her goods in pounds, shillings and pence. A pound was worth 20 old shillings (s.) and a shilling was worth 12 old pence (d) and there were also halfpennies as well as quarter-pennies known as farthings. Some prices, especially for horses, were given in guineas (1 guinea was 21 shillings), and probate inventories tended to use the medieval unit of a mark (13s. 4d) and fractions of it.

Throughout the day Samuel sent his clerks with messages – he needed his black gown, there was a document he had left behind, he was dining in one of the colleges where he was registrar, could Sarah order some sack from Owen Mayfield as he was entertaining the other aldermen in the evening. Supper was taken at about six in the evening, and was usually bread, cheese or cold meat, with wine, sugar cakes and tobacco pipes for visitors who called in afterwards.

Sarah attended civic dinners and observed civic ceremonies, and her friends must have included the wives of other aldermen, who would have had a number of items of news and gossip to compare. There is no evidence of how she spent her spare time, if she had any, or if she could read, but she could probably add up household bills and do accounts. It is women like Sarah who are hidden from history, partly because they had no legal identity, but it is was clearly a happy marriage, for it lasted fifty-seven years, and although it must have had the usual irritations of married life, these were negligible.

One source of irritation for Sarah might have been the Christmas during Samuel's mayoral year, when Sarah and her maid stood in the kitchen and must have looked at each other in bewilderment. Every surface was covered with fish and meat, and Samuel was at the door, a notebook in his hand, beaming as each gift arrived. The first knock at the door was from Mr Jacob who brought six bottles of sack and a sugar loaf; he was followed by the servant of Newton's near neighbour Mrs Sarah Simpson with a keg of sturgeon. Two more sturgeon arrived from William Hinton, who added six bottles of wine, and Mr Turner of Butter Row sent another six bottles. Alderman Herring sent two geese, a turkey and the unusual gift of potatoes, while Alderman Tifford sent a whole sheep.

Newton's fellow public notary Richard Pettit came with two turkeys and six bottles of wine, and Newton's friend Nathaniel Crabbe sent a turkey, six mallard and other wildfowl. A collar of brawn arrived from Alderman Murrinder, 12 bottles of sack and six of claret from Alderman Low, and to Sarah's horror and Samuel's delight the gifts continued. By the end of the day they had received 96 bottles of claret, 63 bottles of sack, 12 bottles of unspecified wine, 13 turkeys, five pieces of sturgeon, two geese, six mallard, three collars of brawn, two joints of port, a chine of mutton, a chine of veal, a whole sheep, a sugar loaf and a sack of potatoes.[15]

It was up to Sarah and her maid to do something with the gifts. The bottles could be stored in the buttery, and the sugar loaf was a welcome addition to the store cupboard, but they were not too sure what to do about the potatoes, and how were they going to deal with thirteen turkeys and a whole sheep with head, tail and feet that needed butchering. None of this was Samuel's concern; he knew the meat would come in very useful for the feasts he would give during the rest of his mayoralty.

The fish could be pickled in brine and vinegar, or salted down, and the pork could be salted down, but did the mallards and the poultry come ready plucked and cleaned or was this another job for Sarah and her maid? Suffolk and Norfolk were famous for their turkeys, with flocks of up to a thousand birds sent on foot to the London market. The absence of chicken and venison from the list suggests that chicken were too humble to give as a status gift. Venison was usually a gift passed between the crown and the nobility, or the nobility and the gentry, so the presents tell us something about the diet and expectations of the middling sort like Samuel Newton. Meat, it was clear, was the main feature of the diet, and was seen as an acceptable gift, as was sturgeon, but we might wonder what Alderman Herring was thinking about when he sent potatoes. No seventeenth-century recipes have yet been found for potatoes, although by the eighteenth century there were recipes for boiled, fried and mashed potatoes as well as for potatoes made into cakes and puddings.[16] It was probably the potatoes that gave Sarah Newton the biggest headache that Christmas.

Samuel and Sarah Newton are typical representatives of the elite of Cambridge town's society. Nathaniel Crabbe and his wife mirror the Newtons' experience, with Nathaniel acting as town treasurer and serving as an alderman; entertaining Samuel Newton and the corporation with sugar cakes, white claret and sack. When Crabbe was mayor Newton sent him a Westphalia ham, two capons, and a turkey for Christmas; so Mrs Crabbe was as familiar as Mrs Newton with the irritations of that season.

The Newtons had a large house and only one surviving child. Thomas Manesty, a tailor who lived in St Michael's parish, had a two-roomed house and five children to keep. His front room opened off the street and here he worked sewing ready-to-wear leather leggings, which his wife sold from a stall set up in front of their house. She cooked over the hearth in the room which served both as Thomas's workshop and as the family's living quarters. Their belongings were sparse: a cauldron to hang over the fire, a jug for ale, beakers, and knives and wooden platters which they shared, stools for the family to sit on round the fire, a small table that was Thomas's cutting-out table and where his wife Elizabeth prepared the food, and straw pallet beds in the attic where they slept. Their lifestyle was basic but they were well clothed, usually in garments made of leather patchwork, offcuts from Thomas's leggings (the leggings sold well having a good reputation with agricultural labourers in the country-side for keeping legs dry), and they never went hungry. Their breakfast was usually wholemeal or rye bread, purchased from the baker, washed down with small beer, and their dinner was pottage of which the main ingredient was barley, with scraps of meat, onions and carrots added. This was on the go all the time, and reappeared with bread for supper as a soup. For a special treat, when funds were good, one of the children would either be sent to a nearby cook shop to fetch rolls filled with meat and laced with mustard, or to a confectioner to buy some sugar cakes.[17]

The poor could have none of these treats. They were dependent on parish relief and alms given out by the colleges. In 1666 George Brierley, his wife and six children were living in a small cottage in Jesus Lane, in All Saints parish, but his parish of legal settlement, which he could apply to for poor relief, was St Botolph's. It was to the churchwardens and overseers of the poor for that parish, Thomas Dawney, William Dickinson, James Stukeley and Edward Morris, that he applied in 1665 when he could not find any work and his family faced starvation. He was given 1s. 4d a week, which he supplemented by sending his children out to beg, and his wife to look for alms from the colleges. Their pottage was mostly water flavoured with such wild herbs as could be found in the hedgerows, and often eaten cold when they could not afford fuel for their fire. Bread was a luxury, and their clothes were threadbare. George tried to make sure that his children ate, and as a result of this privation in January 1666 when the weather was at its worst, he fell seriously ill. As he lay dying the overseers stepped in and sent Thomas Denford's wife to nurse him. They gave the family 6s. 4d for provisions, and when he died they paid 9s. for his burial, including 2d spent on tolling the passing bell. His wife and four of his children were to die of the plague in July 1666, and they were buried in All Saints parish.[18]

College society mirrored the hierarchical character of town society. At the apex of the college pyramid was the master or president of the college. He was the only married member of the academic staff, and had his own house or lodge, and his own servants. When Edward Morton, president of Queens' College died in 1662 he left an estate of £312 9s. 8d, placing him in the same economic bracket as professional men such as Samuel Newton but below that of Richard Pettit, another public notary, who left an estate worth £470 17s. 10d. John Howarth, master of Magdalene College who died in 1668, had an estate worth £220 10s. His lodge consisted of eight rooms. On the first floor was the 'upper room', the chapel chamber and the grooms' chamber, and at ground level next to the street the men's chamber, the hall, a study and a closet adjoining the study. The men's chamber looked back to the custom of tutor and students rooming together which was becoming obsolete by the late seventeenth century.[19]

Below the master but with an equal voice in the governance of the college were the fellows. They were the college equivalent of landed society, aristocracy or gentry as much of their stipend came from the rents of the colleges' endowed estates, and from livings and curacies. Ordained fellows preferred livings within a morning's ride from Cambridge so that they could continue to live in their colleges. Forty pounds a year was considered a good stipend for a fellow in the 1660s.

Fourteen probate inventories exist for college fellows for the period 1661–66. These range from goods worth £778 15s. owned by Edward Stearne, a fellow of Pembroke College, to £4 for John Hodge, a fellow of Sidney Sussex College. However, Edward Stearne had debts amounting to £1,551 12s. 8½d, although £690 in ready money was discovered hidden around his rooms. The two lutes and a bass viol included in the inventory of his goods were later found not to belong to him. Stearne had been expelled from the college in the Parliamentarian purge of 1646; before he left he scratched a message on the window of one of his rooms on the first floor of Ivy Court, expressing his love for the college. He was back after the Restoration, and complaints appeared in the college records about the expense of resettling him.[20]

The value of a fellow's goods may reflect his college stipend, or may indicate access to private funds, or personal preference about what he spent his money on, and how he wanted to live. There was no uniformity even within colleges; for example, Stephen Hall, a fellow of Jesus College who died in 1661, had goods worth £306 18s. 8d, whereas William Davy, a fellow of the same college who died in December 1666, had goods valued at £24 14s. 6d.[21] As might be expected, books made up a significant proportion of the inventories' value.

The inventories tell us something about how the fellows lived. William Baudin of Corpus Christi, who died in 1663, lived in an unheated bed-sitting room crowded with beds and bedding, chairs and a table, and surrounded by books. Robert Beverley of Gonville and Caius College also lived in a bed-sitting room, but he had a fireplace, and added some luxuries – a couch, a looking-glass, wall hangings – and he owned a gold ring. John Boult from the same college had two rooms, a lower chamber with chairs, a couch and a fireplace, and an upper room where he slept, and his luxuries included a silver tobacco box, two gold rings and a silver spoon.[22] How fellows furnished their rooms was up to them, but when the rooms were vacated or exchanged the college took an inventory of immoveable items such as doors, door hinges, locks and keys, windows, fixed shelves and desks.[23]

The next level of college society was that of the commoners, sons of wealthy families, heirs to great estates and putative courtiers. They came to Cambridge to be 'finished' and to meet and make influential friends and connections; many of them had no interest in learning but preferred to hunt, gamble, race their horses, fish and go boating.[24] There were of course exceptions to this: some young noblemen embraced scholarship, and all potential courtiers and politicians found that arguing against false claims in disputation was useful in later life. Finally, there were the minor gentry like Isaac Newton, sons of professional men, merchants and tradesmen of all sorts; some of them had scholarships or bursaries; others, like Newton who entered

Trinity College in 1660, acted as sizars who paid for their keep by helping out fellows or wealthier students, doing secretarial jobs, running errands and performing domestic tasks such as lighting fires. Newton was Dr Babington's sizar, and as Babington was frequently absent from college, his duties were not too onerous.[25]

Isaac Newton had to share a room in college, and this was not a happy arrangement, as John Conduit's collection of papers on Newton shows.[26] John Wickens, who eventually became Newton's room-mate, met him one day in 'the Walks', where he found Newton 'solitary and dejected'. Wickens thought Newton 'disagreeable'; however, they fell into conversation, the result of which was that they agreed to room together. It is debatable whether Newton was a more agreeable room-mate for Wickens than his previous companion. Newton stayed up until two or three in the morning conducting chemical experiments, and often nearly burned the place down by going out and leaving candles alight, and he admitted that one of his sins was 'Denying my chamber fellow of the knowledge that I took him for a drunken sot'.[27]

What might have been immediately obvious to a visitor from today to a college in the 1660s was the youth of the college community. The average age of fellows was 22, so they were barely a few years older than their students, who by the latter half of the seventeenth century were aged between 16 and 17.[28]

Colleges were a society of men, and life could be volatile both within the college and with other colleges and the town. Broken windows and broken heads were often the result, and the proctors, the university's police force, roamed the town at night to apprehend badly behaved students and arrest women of easy virtue who might lead them astray. The proctors raided taverns in the centre of town and brothels in the west of the town to rout out wrongdoers. The proctors themselves were fellows of colleges, and left the rough work to their men. Philip Chapman, a 'proctor's man' died in August 1665.

He lived in a four-roomed house in Little St Mary's parish, and each room was crammed with possessions. On the first floor was the 'Drum Chamber' where there was a bed and bedding, a long table, six chairs, a form, a sideboard, a striped carpet, and a basket and chest. Next to this room was the Fore Chamber, with two beds and bedding in it and a number of 'old' chairs. Downstairs was a parlour and the hall, which was the main living space in the house, and contained a pine table, six rush chairs, eleven pewter dishes, three pewter flagons, four chamber pots, brass cooking implements, a tin colander and a tin dripping pan, two spits, a gridiron, tongs and a fire shovel. The whole was valued at £12 1s. 1d.[29]

The colleges could not have operated without a large domestic staff, although not all were full-time or permanent. The butler, chief cook and porter were usually on a stipend, and some colleges also retained a baker, barber and gardener. Other staff were hired on a casual basis as needed, while much of the maintenance work was done by outside contractors.[30]

The college porter, guardian of the college gates, was an important figure. Usually dressed in college livery, he was the first person a visitor encountered. In the seventeenth century most porters lived outside the college, but close by, for example Ellis Sutton the porter of Peterhouse. However, Edmund Bailey, porter of Christ's College, lived in one room on college premises which might have been the equivalent of the porter's lodge.[31]

Another important figure was the butler. James Coates, the butler of Pembroke College, who died in May 1665, lived outside the college, but close to it in a tall thin house with five rooms. On its ground floor were the hall and kitchen. The kitchen included cooking utensils and a chair for a child. Beneath the hall was a cellar containing beer, a silver bowl, two silver spoons and the valuable household linen. Over the hall were two bedchambers.[32]

The college cook was an essential part of the college. He was paid a stipend of at least £20 a year. The inventories of seven college cooks exist for the period 1663–70, and these show that a college cook could be a very wealthy man. William Cobham the cook of Sidney Sussex College and who died in July 1663 left his granddaughter Ann Stacey £60 and two silver beer bowls, two silver wine cups, one silver gilt salt and a large amount of pewter, as well as a lease from the Dean and Chapter of Ely worth £100. The estate valuations of other college cooks – John Danks of Peterhouse, Thomas Gibbs of Magdalene, William Grimbaud of Queens' and John Howell of Emmanuel – were all worth between £40 and £50 when they died.[33] As well as being college cooks some, such as William Gibson of Magdalene College, also ran a cook shop and lived above it. By contrast, John Howell, the cook of Emmanuel College, lived in a large detached house with nine rooms and a yard where he kept pigs, close to the college. His goods included two bibles, two Common Prayer books, and a book of ethics.[34]

College kitchens demanded a great deal of labour. Apart from the college cook, who was in an executive position, there were specialists in sauces, pastry and sweetmeats, as well as unskilled labour: scullions, kitchen porters, boys to turn spits, servitors and waiters. Extra help was hired in for college feasts and other great occasions.

Some colleges employed their own baker, while others leased out their bakehouse. St John's College paid its baker £8 a year in the 1660s (by the nineteenth century this had risen to £140 a year). Thomas Peck was the baker at Trinity College, and Nicholas Goldsborough at Clare College. When Goldsborough died in May 1666 his goods were worth £57 16s. 2d. They included pictures of the King and Queen as well as other pictures, and the tools of his trade – a kneading trough, skimmer, boulting tub and wheat.[35]

All of these men would have been well known around town: John Danks, for example, was Inspector of Fish at Stourbridge Fair in 1664.[36] But their position was ambiguous. When contention broke out between town and gown, where did their loyalties lie? With the college where they earned a living or the town where they lived? This was especially true for the college gardeners who were hired on a part-time basis and had other employment in town. Nathaniel Bacon a tailor was also the gardener for Corpus Christi College, Daniel Horton was a victualler and landlord of the Cardinal's Cap Inn as well as the gardener for Pembroke College, and John Crudd was a cordwainer and gardener for Trinity Hall.[37]

The same dilemma may have faced the tradesmen contracted to work on college maintenance, such as Thomas Bunning a labourer who did odd jobs for Gonville and Caius College, or John Westley a mason who worked on various colleges, and left £300 to his wife when he died in 1664 and £100 to each of his children.[38] Other townsmen depended on the colleges to buy their goods. Robert Swan, a vintner who supplied fine wine to the colleges, had £60 worth of Canary and French wine in his cellar when he died in 1667. Printers, stationers and booksellers depended on the university and the colleges for trade. John Field, a printer who died in 1668, left £1,700 worth of stock in his shop, and in 1661 Thomas Moody a bookseller had books valued at £80 waiting to be sold.[39]

It is likely that in the late seventeenth century the concept of loyalty to town or gown did not enter the heads of tradesmen and shopkeepers. They had to earn a living and, provided the colleges paid the going rates for goods and service, they were content to leave partisanship to the more radical members of the town such as the dissenting attorney Bryan Kitchingman, or the town's disaffected youth.

Although colleges were a male society, some women were admitted to work as laundresses and cleaners; and the young women of

Cambridge clamoured to become bed-makers in the hope of catching a wealthy husband. In the 1650s St John's College paid its laundresses £2 18s. 6d for six months' work.[40] Isaac Newton paid his 'woman' Agatha and his bed-maker himself. In 1665, before he left Trinity College due to the plague he paid his laundress 6d and his bed-maker 5s. Goodwife Powell was either his laundress or an agent for laundresses, for he 'Paid Goodwife Powell for my laundress 5s', and when he returned from exile in the country in 1666 he paid her a further 7s. 6d and a further 8s. 6d for the laundress. He also paid 6d to Dr Babington's 'gyp', 6d to the porter and 6d to his own 'gyp'.[41] Gyps did heavy jobs such as carrying goods, brushing muddy clothes, or taking messages. They held the keys to students' rooms, and could report anyone absent overnight.[42]

The colleges needed the townspeople to play many different roles, and the town needed the colleges for employment and to buy goods and services. When the plague closed the university and the colleges, both suffered economically, and some of the individuals described in this chapter were directly affected. Samuel and Isaac Newton left town for the countryside, as did most of the college masters and fellows. Thomas Manesty was to bury his children during the plague, and the Brierley family, who lost their father just before the plague began, was to be decimated by it. College cooks, bakers, laundresses and gyps were out of work during the plague, and only the porters remained to guard the closed doors with their lives.

CHAPTER 4

IMPENDING DISASTER

THE YEAR 1665 started with a great frost. Samuel Pepys noted that on 5 January there was cold, great snow and frost, and that 6 February was one of the coldest days he had ever known.[1] In Essex Ralph Josselin wrote that there was frost from 21 December 1664 until 9 February 1665.[2] In Cambridge, streets and outside stairs became dangerous and slippery. Mr Greswell, a fellow of Trinity College, slipped on icy stairs next to the college chapel and was found dead, cold and still by bed-makers the next morning. It transpired that he had been drinking and was let back into college by the porters at two in the morning, and it was assumed that he had been going to his college rooms from the house of easement in the garden.[3]

Cambridge people huddled in front of their hearths, or went out bundled up in their warmest clothes. Their breath hung on the icy air. Apothecaries sold great quantities of salve for chilblains, prepared from betony, figwort, hyssop or kidney wort, either made into an ointment with honey and lard, or distilled into water to bathe the itching blains.[4] Feet were wrapped in rags to ease the pressure of shoes, and country people coming into town beat their blains with holly to make them bleed and relieve the itching.[5] Faces were red and chapped. Bruised pennyroyal could ease this, or lovage fried in hog's lard and applied as a salve.[6] Prudent mothers sewed their children into vests coated with fat for the duration, to keep them warm and cosy and prevent winter chills.

In the streets medicinal smells mingled with those from cook shops that were doing a literally roaring trade as frozen citizens thawed out beside their hearths. After dark, which came early in the winters of seventeenth-century Cambridge, the streets were black and deserted, lit only by a few lamps hung out by householders, and flaming torches held by link men leading fellows to their colleges, scholars to public houses, or members of the corporation on their way home from the Three Tuns tavern, where they had been after the funeral of Mrs Susanna Wells.[7] It was a land of black and white and shadows, surrounded by a sea of frozen fens.

The thaw began on 14 March, turning roads into rivers, and the River Cam into a torrent racing through Cambridge and threatening the bridges. Despite this, life slowly returned to normal. March 16 1665 was the corporation's audit day, which was followed by a 'very good dinner', and on 24 March the corporation, as was the tradition, went fishing, 'as many aldermen as pleased'; common council men, the mayor, town recorder and treasurers went fishing on the Cam in three hired boats. They drew first at Newnham pond, and then at the mills, and fished down the river to 'Bullins', where they had the fish they had caught dressed and partook of bread, cheese and wine, for an overall cost of £5.[8]

Also in March another great procession came into town when the assizes led by the circuit judge Lord Keeling arrived to stay at Trinity College. Here the town's treasurers and representatives of the butchers and fishmongers went to wait on him. They were ushered into the college's kitchens where the gifts to the judge from the mayor and corporation were displayed: a veal, a sheep, a pike, two ducks, two eels and six perch. The judge refused to see the representatives from the corporation, but his steward told them he would pass on the corporation's greetings and tell His Lordship about the presents. The master and scholars of Trinity College presented the judge with a pair of embroidered gloves worth 30s., which they were allowed to present to him in person.[9]

The difference in the gifts made to the judge by the corporation and the college, both bestowed in the hope of favours in the future, illustrates the different mindsets of the two. Corporation life was punctuated by refreshments and dinners, so the corporation had provided what they thought would be most useful to the judge – a supply of victuals; hence the college's gift of gloves was an acknowledgement of the judge's position and they got to meet the judge, while the corporation's representatives did not. This was all part of the hierarchical nature of seventeenth-century society and the rivalry between the colleges and the town, but the corporation was also shunned because of the town's part in the Civil War; it was only two years since the corporation had been purged of its Parliamentarians and members who had refused to swear allegiance to the king. As the king's representative, the judge may have considered that it was still inappropriate to acknowledge the corporation as an official body.

The assizes were held in Cambridge Castle and Samuel Newton attended. The cases tried included robbery, murder and slighting words against the Lord Chief Justice. John Patteson was sentenced to stand in the pillory from 11.15 to 12.30 for the crime of 'barratry', the misdemeanour of provoking or maintaining lawsuits or quarrels in order to keep lucrative cases in court.[10]

One unfortunate, Edward Sterne, was known to Newton as he was apprenticed to Newton's 'brother Woolley'. Sterne was charged with the robbery of Mr Marden, but refused to plead and was sentenced to be 'pressed to death, which was done between 5–7 in the afternoon: He took an hour to die, at his pressing he confessed himself guilty of this and other robberies.'[11] Pressing was a horrible death as the victim was laid on the ground and stones piled on him until he was crushed. Newton witnessed this and two hangings.[12]

Despite the snow and ice of the winter months, following the thaw there was no rain, and by 9 April the threat of a drought.[13] By that time England was at war with the Dutch. The rivalry with Holland was over trade and the freedom of the seas. Both nations were eager to expand their colonies and markets and to exploit the spice islands of the East Indies and the slave markets of Africa. A national fast to aid the Dutch War by prayer was proclaimed for 5 April and observed in Cambridge.[14]

A day later the war came to Cambridge directly when the press-gang arrived to take men to serve on the ships. 'Some 3 or 4 score men [60–80] were taken, including John Sparkes, the son of John Sparkes the baker.'[15] John Sparkes was one of Samuel Newton's neighbours and had baptised a daughter, Mary, in 1656. The names of the other men taken are not known, but it is likely that few returned. Like John Sparkes they would have been young men, with young families who were left to fend for themselves. However, John Sparkes did return from the war, and lived to a good age, making his will in 1683. He left his daughter Mary £30 to be paid to her when she reached the age of thirty-five provided she did not marry Charles Browne, a bookseller of Cambridge. If she married him she was to have only 1s. Similarly, he left his son John 1s., but also the willow trees in Sheep Cote, and all John's debts to his father were remitted. The will was witnessed by Samuel Newton.[16]

As well as the men pressed into service in Cambridge, a further 400 men were assembled in the town from the countryside, ready to join the fleet at Harwich.[17] The fleet consisted of 190 vessels, some of them great purpose-built warships, but ill equipped and badly provisioned. The men from Cambridge would never have seen the sea or been on a ship before. Seasickness was rife, as prevailing easterlies buffeted the ships. Many men were lost overboard: they fell from the rigging, slipped on the damp decks, or threw themselves into the sea from sheer desperation. They were untrained, and unready to go to war.

On 3 June the men from Cambridge saw action for the first time, and the pounding of the guns in the North Sea could be heard in the town. 'Saturday all day long was heard the noise of guns in the air and between 4 and 6 in the afternoon and again between 9 and 10 the same night, it was generally thought at Cambridge that the Dutch and English had engaged,' wrote Samuel Newton in his diary.[18] The engagement off the Suffolk coast became known as the Battle of Lowestoft, and it was inconclusive. The English lost one ship, but failed to capitalise on the Dutch retreat. Despite this on 20 June there was a public thanksgiving for an English victory.[19] The war would continue at sea, but by the end of June 1665 the country had other things on its mind. Plague had been confirmed in London, Portsmouth and Great Yarmouth,[20] and the war faded into the background.

It was not unexpected. The conjunction of the stars, the appearance of a comet, and the exceptionally cold weather were all portents of an impending disaster. Now it was clear what this disaster entailed.

Apprehension and anxiety about the pestilence led to panic. Once the cry of plague went up, people began to see plague spots everywhere – on walls, gates and doors, on animals and in the sky.[21] Social prejudices emerged. The plague was the fault of the Dutch, the French, the drunks, the lechers or the misfits in society. The poor were blamed: because they lived in overcrowded, dirty and unhygienic houses the plague must be their fault for allowing these conditions to exist; and if the plague was caused by Man's sinfulness, then the poor must be especially sinful.[22]

Cambridge was one of the wealthier towns in the country. The university helped to provide full employment and there was plenty of opportunity for trade and temporary jobs at Stourbridge Fair, but there were pockets of poverty in the town and 14 per cent of the householders listed in the Cambridge Hearth Tax were too poor to pay the tax.[23]

Travellers and carriers coming from London confirmed that plague was present in the capital city. The news caused a sick jolt to the stomach and nauseous feeling in the throat. Waiting for the plague was the worst thing. Every little pimple and insect bite meant the plague, every high body temperature meant panic. Was this the plague? Neighbour eyed neighbour with suspicion. Was that spot on the nose a plague token? Were closed shutters the sign of a stricken household? As the heat of the summer grew, so did the fear of plague.

The Cambridge carriers William Waterson, Roger Hurst, Thomas Morrow and John Styles[24] began to bring in the London Bills of Mortality, which showed the progress of the plague. These were prudently hung in the air before anyone dared read them.

On 21 June Samuel Pepys saw confusion at the Cross Keys at Cripple Gate, as almost all who could were fleeing in coaches and wagons, and by July 1665 there were complaints in Hertfordshire about the refugees from London flooding into the county bringing infection with them.[25] Towns closed their gates and set watches to stop Londoners entering, so they were forced to camp in the surrounding fields.

The summer heat intensified. The river level in Cambridge dropped, leaving banks of decaying slime which added to the stench of the dunghills and garbage in the streets. The townspeople wiped the sweat from their brows, every window and door was flung open,

and naked children played in the streets, while the elderly sat and
fanned themselves in the shade, and swatted flies. Those flies – no
one had ever seen so many flies, getting in the hair, up the nose, in
the mouth and settling on food. 'A multitude of flies that lived on the
inside of houses, and swarms of ants covering highways, winged and
creeping,' wrote William Boghurst in a passage reminiscent of the
plagues of Egypt.[26]

The cook shops doused their fires, fishmongers closed up and
butchers cut back on their stock. Meat, fish, fruit and vegetables
rotted in the heat.

The nights were the worst. Children whimpered, unable to sleep,
bed covers were thrown off, every window was left unshuttered and
open. Just a breath of air was savoured like a draught of best wine.
Cambridge sweltered in the heat, and every day the sun shone down
from a cloudless sky when the town longed for grey skies and rain to
damp down the dust in the streets, bring life to the parched grass on
college lawns, and sweeten the air.

Tension in Cambridge grew. The town and the colleges were
waiting . . . waiting for something to happen, holding their collective
breath. Then on 25 July 1665 they knew. The plague had arrived and
claimed its first victim. This was little John Morley. On the same day
as John Morley's little brother died in the pest house, Anne the small
daughter of John Fisher, died of the plague in All Saints parish. It
was spreading through the streets.[27]

Where had the plague come from? The corporation had already
enforced the Privy Council's Plague Orders, and strangers were only
allowed into town with a certificate of health. The streets were
cleansed and stray dogs and cats killed. The pest houses were ready,
and the searchers who identified the plague victims were hired.[28]
Surely everything had been done to prevent the sickness? The first
three victims were little children, who could not be held responsible

for the sins of mankind, but the next victim, Rose Banks of Holy Trinity who died in the pest house on 10 August 1665, was probably no better than she should have been. The daughter of Thomas and Elizabeth Banks, she had been baptised on 28 October 1605 and so in terms of the life expectancy of the seventeenth century was old; by the time of her death she had had a long and chequered career. One of a large family, she had ten brothers and sisters, and as the eldest girl was the carer for her younger siblings from an early age, especially as her mother had a child every year between 1604 and 1616.[29] Everyone, or rather every man, in Holy Trinity parish knew Rose, while every woman called her a slut, as despite what might be considered a life of drudgery Rose managed to have a good time. She was often seen serving in the Unicorn in Petty Cury, or drinking in one of the other inns, and part of her good time was going with handsome lads and married men who took her fancy, sometimes in the long grass at the bottom of King's College Field, and once on a winter's evening under a stall in the Market Place.[30] The result of these exploits was that she baptised two illegitimate sons, one of whom was buried in Holy Trinity churchyard in 1644.[31] Despite her moral failings, Rose Banks was much missed around town.

Other residents in Holy Trinity parish were Ellen and Richard Lawrence who had moved into the parish in 1663, taking over a house vacated by John Else. He was one of the town's inhabitants who desperately hoped that Stourbridge Fair would not be cancelled, as, despite being fined for selling false measures of beer at Midsummer and Stourbridge Fairs,[32] he knew he could make a good living at these fairs with very little effort. Neighbours told the Lawrences that John Else was a 'bit of a lad' who had got Mary Mitchell into trouble.[33]

Goody Ellen Lawrence did not worry about the previous tenant's reputation. This was a good solid house, with a hall and kitchen on the ground floor, each with a hearth, and a loft area. At the back was a communal yard, which in earlier days had been laid out as garden plots, but now, because of the demand for housing in Cambridge, had been in-filled with cottages leaving just a small open space.[34] Washing could be hung here, there was a communal house of office (toilet), and Ellen grew a small patch of herbs by her back door. The neighbours were decent as well. Samuel Frohock who lived in a larger house next door was a butcher with stalls in the Shambles, and William Russell on the other side was an upright man.[35] A year after they moved into the cottage in Holy Trinity, the Lawrences were blessed with a little girl, baptised Sarah on 3 January 1664, a playmate for the next-door neighbour's three-year-old son John Frohock.[36]

When her husband came home complaining of a headache, Ellen was not unduly worried. It was the heat. She brewed him a soothing drink of camomile in hot water and sent him to bed, and then sat in the evening sun nursing Sarah. At one point she heard her husband cry out, and found him shivering and calling for water. During the night she could not sleep because he was thrashing about and muttering, and when she got up and lit a candle she saw that her husband's eyes were staring and his mouth was open in a grimace of pain. In the flickering light she saw swellings in his groin and armpits – there was no doubt Richard had the plague. She sat by him all night, then reluctantly, because she was a good citizen she sent for the searchers within the two-hour window specified in the town's Plague Orders.[37] She spent the little time she had before the house was closed gathering as many herbs as she could, and passing a few coins in a bowl of vinegar out to her neighbours in the hope that they would buy her food and other necessities. Her house became her prison. Richard died on 11 August 1665.[38] Forty days later Ellen emerged blinking into the sunlight with Sarah in her arms. She would not tell of the horrors she had experienced, but packed up her belongings and left, wanting to escape the house of death for ever.

As the plague took a firm hold on Cambridge the university was closed, the college gates clanged shut, and fellows and scholars were given leave of absence. At Jesus College, which was closed on 7 August 1665, three fellows voluntarily stayed at their posts,[39] but most colleges had rural manors close to Cambridge, where fellows could move during the plague outbreak and maintain a society similar to that in college. Other fellows went to the homes of their students or wealthy patrons.[40] Not all fellows deserted their colleges. One stayed on in Clare College and sent out news of the progress of the plague in Cambridge to friends in London.[41] William Bunchley, the manciple (quartermaster) of Christ's College stayed at his post and died of the plague, prompting a wholesale flight from the college.[42] John Francius, a fellow of Peterhouse was too sick too travel and died on 21 June 1665, while Theodore Crosland, senior fellow of Trinity College, and Walter Costry also of Trinity stayed on: both died in September, but there was no mention of the plague in connection with their deaths.[43]

One scholar who departed was Isaac Newton, who was a student at Trinity College in 1665, and returned home to Woolsthorpe in Lincolnshire. In old age he told his niece's husband John Conduit, who was collecting material to write Newton's life, 'that it was while in exile at Woolsthorpe that he discovered his system of gravity, the first hint of it coming when he saw a loose apple fall from a tree . . .'[44]

Stourbridge Fair was cancelled by royal proclamation on 7 August 1665. The town was securely in the grip of the plague.

CHAPTER 5

THE INFECTED SUMMER

IN THAT SUMMER of 1665 the riverside parish of St Clement had a smell all of its own: rotting vegetation on the riverbank and from the ooze of black mud where the river had dried up, mingled with the sweet malt smell from Thompson's Brewery. The King's Ditch re-entered the river here, and passers-by noticed and shuddered at the great number of dead rats lying around the ditch. The houses in St Clement's were crowded together in courts, alleys and yards, and Bridge Street was one of the busiest streets in Cambridge. Shops, inns and the parish church fronted it, and it was always thronged with shoppers buying meat from James Wendy's butcher's shop, bread from John Hill's bakery or drapery from Widow Linsey, or stopping for a drink at one of its many inns.[1]

A group of teenagers who lived in the parish were firm friends, and spent as much time as possible together. In summer, when their elders allowed them some free time, they went to Jesus Green to kick a leather ball about or, if it was too hot, to lie in the long grass by the river to banter and gossip, and share a jug of ale or a pipe of tobacco.

On Jesus Green was a number of timber-framed huts set in a compound with a strong fence and a padlocked gate. The teenagers accepted these as part of the scenery; a few even squeezed through the fence to look inside, and reported that the huts were like empty houses, and some even had beds in them, a fact stored away for the future as a place where a girl could be taken for some privacy.

Earlier in the year there had been activity in the sheds. Holes in the roofs were repaired, the wattle and daub walls had been lime-washed and stouter padlocks added to all the doors. The teenagers and children of St Clement's were told to stay way from Jesus Green on pain of a severe beating. The huts were pest houses being prepared for an epidemic of plague. Banned from Jesus Green, the teenagers took to congregating by the Great Bridge, where they could watch travellers arriving in town and perhaps earn a few pennies holding horses or directing people to local inns.

One of the teenagers on the bridge was Jacob, aged 14, the son of Francis King a tailor and his wife Jane. The Kings had lived in St Clement's parish since 1646, and had buried two children in the parish churchyard, Alice aged two in 1648 and Francis, also aged two, in 1655, followed by their mother Jane in 1658, so that Jacob and his father were left to fend for themselves. Jacob ran wild until the parish overseers of the poor took him in hand and apprenticed him to David Bowen, a shoemaker.[2] It took Jacob some time to get used to the discipline of work, but in 1665 with only a few years left of his apprenticeship he looked forward to becoming a journeyman and setting up on his own. When his friends asked him what he did, he leered and said he measured the feet of pretty ladies, but really he found great satisfaction in cutting out leather to exact measurements and creating a shoe which would last for years.

On the evening of Sunday 13 August the young people gathered on the bridge as usual.[3] They included the Pawston brothers, Daniel,

Samuel and Luke, and their big sister Alice aged 15, Jennet Bird aged 13, her 11-year-old brother John and their little sister Ann aged seven; with them was Ann Austin, a mystery girl who had moved into the parish recently with her father Robert.[4]

It had been another exceptionally hot and sunny day. In the morning the group on the bridge had been to the parish church, as they were obliged to do, and had taken part in prayers for those visited by the sickness in Cambridge and London. Now they had a few hours of liberty before starting work on the Monday morning.

They were all brown as nuts from the sun, but Jacob King's face was unnaturally red and he rubbed discontentedly at a red spot on his arm. A flea bite, he supposed. He decided he had had enough for one day and would visit his father and spend the night with him, as it would be a relief to get away from Bowen's 19-year-old bully of a son, Thomas.[5]

Usually Jacob would have run home, but this time he walked because his legs felt heavy. He found his father sitting at the front door of his house which doubled as his tailor's workshop. Jacob walked through the workshop to the kitchen at the back to get a drink of small ale from an earthenware jug standing in a bowl of water to keep it cool. A small spit and fire jack stood in the empty hearth, with a kettle beside it, and a warming pan hung nearby. There were a table and bench, some wooden platters, a bowl and knife on a hanging shelf. It was not luxurious, but it was comfortable. In a chamber up a short flight of stairs was his father's wooden bed with its rope base and feather mattress, bolster and an old sheet, and beneath the bed was a pull-out trundle bed, which Jacob pulled out and lay on.[6] When his father came up to see if he would like some bread and cheese, Jacob vomited.

Francis King looked at his son, whose face was burning, and decided to take some of his small hoard of cash and buy lotion from Peter Dent the apothecary who lived just across the road, in a house that backed on to Holy Sepulchre church (the Round Church). Dent sold Francis a lotion of distilled water made from the leaves and flowers of borage, grown in Dent's physic garden.[7] Borage not only helped to reduce fever, but in the seventeenth century was also thought to reduce melancholy and depression, and melancholy was seen as a symptom of plague.[8]

It was during the 1665–66 plague that the trade of the apothecary became recognised as an honourable profession, as they stayed put while physicians fled from infected towns and cities. Apothecaries served a seven-year apprenticeship in which they learned about diseases, symptoms, and potions to help the sufferer. At the end of his apprenticeship the apothecary set up shop and not only sold medicines but also traded in other commodities such as dried fruit, tobacco, thread and oils.

There were five apothecaries in Cambridge during the 1665–66 plague outbreak. As well as Peter Dent there was Alderman Artemus Hinde who lived in St Giles parish, William Frisby and Martin Buck, friends of Samuel Newton, and Charles Gilman. Of these, Peter Dent was the most distinguished. A native of Cambridge born in 1629 he attended Trinity College between 1649 and 1650. It is not known where he served his apprenticeship, but he set up his own shop in Bridge Street in 1657. He was involved in town affairs, acting as inspector of tobacco at Stourbridge Fair in 1656, 1660 and 1667, and at Midsummer Fair in 1659. When he died in 1689 he was described in his will as an apothecary and Reader of Physic, having been given a licence to practise as a physician 'on recommendation'. He left his business to his son Pierce and asked him to keep on his apprentice William Smith for his full term.[9]

Apothecaries needed a working knowledge of Latin and a good knowledge of plants as most of their remedies were herb based. Some of these might soothe the plague patient, but none could cure.

During the night Jacob fell into an uneasy sleep, sometimes shuddering or crying out.[10] The buboes appeared in his armpits. There was no doubt that it was the plague. On 15 August 1665 Jacob died. He was the first plague victim in St Clement's. As the bell tolled for his passing, so news spread through the streets. Francis King was shut up in the house of death, and no one followed Jacob's body to the churchyard, although as it passed the almshouses Widows Walker and Lamb whispered prayers for his soul. Plague victims in Cambridge had to be buried before sun-rising or after sun-setting, and no friends or neighbours were allowed to attend, enter the house of the dead, or gawp at the corpse from a doorway.[11]

As Jacob lay dying, Cambridge corporation decided to cancel the dinner to mark the election of a new mayor, and the Cambridge Bills of Mortality started to appear fortnightly from 10 August 1665 onwards. The Bill for 10–25 August 1665 recorded seventeen burials in the town of which five were of plague victims.[12] Samuel Newton received the London Bills of Mortality for 15–22 August, and laboriously copied the figures into his diary. 'Buried within the walls 538, whereof of plague buried 366. Buried in the 16 parishes without the walls of plague 2139.'[13]

On 24 August the corporation rather belatedly ordered that 'in regard to information that plague is in every parish in the kingdom, for sundry measures in this town, all public meetings are banned'.[14] This meant that the election of a new mayor was cancelled, along with the civic festivities that would have accompanied it.

The incubation period for the plague was 2–6 days after exposure, but it could be as long as 10–12 days; while death could take place within 1–2 days, some lingered in pain for much longer.[15] The next two plague victims in St Clement's may have been infected from the same source as Jacob King. Grace, the daughter of Joseph Gilbert, and the mystery girl Ann Austin were both buried on 30 August.[16]

Two days later another of the teenagers on the bridge Daniel Pawston died, on 9 September seven-year-old Ann Bird, and on 13 September Thomas, son of James King.[17]

When Daniel Pawston died of the plague the house where he lived with his family was closed up, the door nailed shut, and the red cross and the words 'Lord Have Mercy Upon Us' painted across it. The house was guarded by watchmen who stood outside day and night to prevent anyone escaping.[18] Inside were Daniel's parents and his brothers and sisters, all suffering from the plague. In the heat of the summer they sweated and cried out for water. The buboes burst on Samuel, Daniel's brother, leaving blood and pus to be cleared up by their already ailing mother, and little Alice Pawston could not breathe and died blue in the face and choking. Samuel died on 15 September, his mother the day after, and the last two Pawston children Luke and Alice on 18 September 1665.

The Pawstons' house was deserted, and it remained empty until after forty days the bedding clothes and soft furnishings were taken out and burned and the house fumigated with limewash and pitch. In later life, Sir Edward Southcote wrote to his son: 'I well remember when I was five years old, the time of the Great Plague of the smoking of the houses with pitch, and the dismal stories that were brought in of people lying dead in the highway that nobody dared bury.'[19] This is corroborated by Samuel Pepys, who recorded in his diary that on 15 August 1665 he saw a plague corpse lying abandoned in an alley, and on the 22nd as he walked to Greenwich that he saw an open coffin, with a plague victim inside it, lying outside a farm.[20]

The Cambridge Bills of Mortality from 7 to 14 September 1665 reported sixteen plague burials of which six were in the pest house, eight in St Clement's parish, and two in the parish of St Andrew the Great.[21] The first two plague deaths in St Andrew's were those of

Jonas Bayley and his three-year-old son George. They lived in a house leased from Jonas's father George, a freeman and burgess of the town, who lived in a substantial house with five hearths in All Saints parish. Jonas had been made a freeman in August 1660, and could look forward to becoming a burgess and leasing a booth at Stourbridge Fair. This was not an impoverished family, and although their occupations are not known, they were in the middle rank of society. Jonas's widow died of the plague on 26 September, leaving George senior to care for baby Alice, aged one year.[22]

St Clement's was fast becoming the epicentre of the plague. By mid-September seven houses were closed and marked with the red cross, and at least one parishioner, Goodwife Bowring, died in the 'old pest house' at Ball's Folly (Lensfield Road); others were in the pest house on Jesus Green, awaiting their fate.

Plague was identified across the river in St Peter's parish as early as August 1665. St Peter's was a small parish with much of its land taken up with pools of stagnant water and willow stands, breeding grounds for mosquito-borne infections, and its houses were mostly poor and crowded together in yards and closes. In particular there were three small houses built into Charles Day's yard, and four families living in one cottage owned by Thomas Mace, the bailiff of Reach Fair and town treasurer.[23]

The churchwardens of St Peter's, Henry Mulliner and William Goodes, were also overseers of the poor. As there were few ratepayers living in St Peter's they had very limited resources, and no option but to send the infected to the pest houses on Jesus Green, where eight unnamed inhabitants of St Peter's parish died in August 1665 and a further twelve in September. Their names are unrecorded; they appear only as numbers in the parish register and their deaths do not appear in the Bills of Mortality. But this parish of about 340 souls in two months lost 6 per cent of its population.[24]

St Giles was one of the two parishes across the River Cam from the town centre. Its houses sprawled up Castle Hill and Castle End, around the castle itself, and beside the church on Chesterton Lane. Cambridge's West Fields edged onto this parish, and the inhabitants of St Giles helped with the harvest in the fields, trudged out in the cold and mud to plough and sow, and sent their children to pick up stones and scare birds from the crops. They could supplement their diet by snaring a rabbit or two on the field, pick blackberries, crab apples and quinces from the hedgerows to turn into preserves, and the more adventurous might venture into the village of Girton to scrump apples and pears, or bag a duck from the Wash Brook.

The inhabitants of St Giles heard the bell tolling across the river in St Clement's, but hoped they might escape infection this time. After all, they reasoned, the parish was self-sufficient, it had its own butcher, baker and fishmonger, and its own apothecary, so if they were careful and people did not wander into town they might be all right. Parents impressed on their children that they should not cross the river or meet their friends on the riverside quay, but they could not keep an eye on them all day long.

St Giles was another poor and overcrowded parish, and here the first plague death took place in a one-roomed hovel which Richard Palmer rented from Mrs Thurlowe. His little daughter Marie died of the plague on 12 September 1665, his two-year-old son Edward on 15 October and his wife Susanna on 15 November. The Palmers had been married in St Giles church on 14 October 1660. From Marie's death to the death of his wife Richard had been shut up in his one room with the dying. He heard the cries of pain, but could do nothing. Pails of water were left for him, and the overseers of the poor left bread, as he had no money to buy provisions. The overseers shook their heads, and muttered that the plague would stretch their resources to the limit.[25]

The plague had settled in St Giles. The next family affected were the Leakes. They were not wealthy, and were bringing up a family of four in a two-roomed cottage on Castle Hill. Robert was a labourer who picked up work where he could, sometimes as a porter on the Quayside and sometimes in the West Fields. When their daughter Alice died from the plague on 21 September, there was an air of resignation about her parents, as if they'd expected this to happen. Alice's brother Robert died on 4 October, and their father a day later, leaving their mother to care for her two surviving children. Their cottage was rented from Thomas Archer, who was not best pleased when it was closed up for forty days and he received no rent.[26]

The infection continued in St Clement's. Nathaniel Aungier who was a lodger in the parish died of the plague and was buried on 27 September 1665, and on the same day John, the son of Henry Gunnell, was buried. Henry Gunnell was the landlord of the Blackamoor's Head, a popular inn on Bridge Street, owned by Peter Lightfoot a local fishmonger and alderman.[27] Closing the inn for forty days meant a loss of revenue for him and a loss of employment for its potmen, cooks, ostlers and servants, as well as loss of trade for those shopkeepers who provided it with beer, bread, meat and cheese. The plague was an economic disaster as well as a tragedy for those who lost loved ones. When Henry Gunnell and his wife came out of quarantine they gave up the inn and moved across the road to St John's Lane, where Henry died in 1667.[28]

The day after John Gunnell was buried, Ann Russell, 'the bastard daughter of Thomas Russell', joined him in the churchyard. Thomas Russell was an innkeeper in St Bene't's parish who was accused by Alice Bradman in 1658 of being the father of her child. He denied this, but as he was known in the town as a lady's man he was made to swear an oath and give a bond to the parish overseers of the poor that he would contribute to the upkeep of the child. He gave Ann his surname and put her out to be fostered with a family in St Clement's.[29]

Harleston Lane was a small twisting lane in the centre of St Clement's, leading off from Bridge Street towards the King's Ditch and Jesus Green. Here there was an enclave of shops and houses, some leased from St John's College and then sublet by John Bullin, a haberdasher.[30] One of his tenants was Luke Horne, who may have come from Wisbech where Horne was a common surname in the seventeenth century. The Horne family tried to avoid going anywhere near the closed-up houses, but to no avail. On 29 September 1665 Mary and Frances, Luke's daughters, aged eight and ten respectively, died of the plague and were buried at the same time as John Stokes, Luke's servant and also a plague victim. Luke's wife Susan was taken away to the pest house on Jesus Green where she died, and Luke was left with one remaining daughter, Susan aged twelve. Luke died two years later, and was buried on 10 May 1668. Susan, left to fend for herself, disappears from the records.[31]

Like the Horne girls, many of those who died in the early stages of the plague in Cambridge were children or teenagers. Statistically there was a strong probability that children would be plague victims, as most households in seventeenth-century England contained children, usually at least two or three. There were children in the houses and children in the streets. Life was undertaken amidst a continual babble of childish voices and childish distractions – demands for food and drink, tears to be mopped up, cuts and grazes to be bathed, arguments to be settled. There were 13 children in the early plague houses in Holy Trinity, 11 in St Andrews' and 30 in six plague houses in St Clement's. When the children died, and their friends were stopped from going outside their houses for fear of infection, silence descended on the streets.

The ubiquity of children and the high infant death rate have led to the conclusion that children were not valued, their deaths were not mourned as those of adults were mourned, and that it was difficult to establish warm personal relationships in the seventeenth century. Infants were often deprived of a mother-figure at an early age, sometimes at birth, so, it is argued, the high death rate for all ages meant that children quickly became wary of placing emotional capital in others. Rage, sensory, physical and emotional deprivation among children created an adult society of emotional cripples, with parents unable to relate to and love their offspring.[32]

This depressing view of seventeenth-century family life has been challenged as a myth, especially as the clergy preached the value of family bonds from the pulpit.[33] Parental love for children is usually innate, and the loss of a child in any century causes parents great suffering and diminishes the family. The more literate members of seventeenth-century society recorded their grief on the death of children. On the death of his five-year-old son Richard, John Evelyn wrote, 'Here ends the joy of my life, which go ever mourning to the grave' and when his daughter Mary died at the age of 19, 'Never can I say enough; oh dear, my dear child, whose memory is so precious.'[34] Ralph Josselin the Essex clergyman of Earl's Colne had ten children, of whom only three survived into adulthood. He recorded his grief for each child. On 21 February 1641 when his baby Ralph died he wrote, 'This day my dear babe Ralph, quietly fell asleep.' A grandmother, Mrs Elizabeth Freke, wrote that when one of her grandchildren died both she and her husband 'were extremely melancholy for the fatal loss of our dear babe'.[35]

Most of the parents in Cambridge who lost children in the plague of 1665–66 could not record their feelings. However, it is possible to track the numbers of children who died and reconstruct some individual families. In the decade before the plague, for the three parishes in Cambridge where there were early plague deaths – All Saints, St Andrew the Great and St Clement's – the burial records show 191 burials in All Saints, of which 30 per cent were children, 187 in St Andrew's (40 per cent children), and 257 in St Clement's (49 per cent children). In St Clement's between 1654 and 1663 fifty-nine families lost children, and some lost more than one. Lewis Covill a baker buried four children; George Skinner and Richard Scarrow and seven other families lost three children each, and a further ten families each lost two children.[36]

But those who could not write down their feelings could, if they were wealthy enough, hire a scrivener or a lawyer to write their wills, and these reveal that, despite the custom by which the eldest son inherited the family estate, land or business, strenuous efforts were made to divide the family assets between all the children. If the wife was pregnant when the will was drawn up, then provision was made for the unborn child.[37] Seventeenth-century wills were couched in legal language, so that the phase 'loving son' or 'loving daughter' might be a legal construct, but to the testator and the beneficiary the phrase may have had real meaning.

Love did not stop parents from chastising their offspring. Slapping or beating a child was not a criminal offence in the seventeenth century. Parents expected obedience from their sons and daughters, and that they keep the commandment, 'Honour thy father and thy mother'. The father ruled the household and his word was law, but the mother ran the household too: she cooked, cleaned and taught her children the way of a good life. Like parents everywhere, the parents in plague-ridden Cambridge wanted the best for their children, and during the plague children were doubly precious.

As September came to a close, the evenings drew in. The mist from the Fens chilled the morning air and the town looked forward to autumn and winter in the hope that the cold would dampen down the plague and allow life to get back to normal.

CHAPTER 6

FALLING LEAVES AND SABLE SKIES

A UTUMN IN CAMBRIDGE was usually an exciting and busy time. The town had cleaned up after Stourbridge Fair; the timber booths were taken down and stored, and the rubbish – tons of it – had been carted away. Shopkeepers, grocers, vintners, butchers and bakers counted their takings and replenished their stock for the coming season. Innkeepers brewed their autumn ale and freshened up their guest rooms: sheets were laundered, bolsters renewed, and furniture polished.

Queues of women waited at the porters' lodges of colleges to see if they would be taken on as bed-makers or laundresses. Domestic bursars allocated rooms to scholars who had returned to Cambridge after the Long Vacation, and college cooks began to plan menus. Not this year. The college gates remained locked, and the colleges brooded over the town in silence and darkness. The university was still closed because of the plague, and there would be no influx of excited young men coming into town with their luggage, calling to each other in the streets, going to lectures, or visiting inns. The college bells would not ring, and their flags and pennants would not fly. There would be no procession of scarlet-clad dons, heralded by the university waits and preceded by mace-bearers, wending their way from the Schools to Great St Mary's church. The bed-makers, kitchen porters and cooks were unemployed, and had to rely on charity for necessities.

Normally in autumn Samuel Newton's civic year progressed with a series of processions, meetings and feasts; the new mayor and aldermen were chosen in September and the corporation went in procession on horseback to the new mayor's house. When Samuel Newton's friend Nathaniel Crabbe was chosen as mayor in 1668, Newton borrowed a horse from Mr Jerman and with other aldermen rode to visit Crabbe at his house at Ball's Folly. Here they alighted and had a cup of sack and a piece of a great cake. They then rode to the old mayor's house, and back to the town hall for dinner: 'we had two dishes of boiled chicken, then a boiled leg of mutton, then a piece of roast beef, then a mutton pasty, then a glass of claret, then two couple of rabbits, then two couple of wild fowl ...' By that time it was two o'clock and the aldermen took off their scarlet gowns and sent for their black gowns and went into the council chamber for a common (business) day. After the meeting Newton and others were invited into the mayor's parlour to take a glass of wine, and 'we had 14 bottles of sack from the Mitre, three quarter pounds of tobacco with pipes, and 3 flagons of beer (as some desired to drink beer)'. Two women had been present at the midday dinner, Mrs Pettit, the wife of the old mayor Richard Pettit, and Mrs Crabbe the wife of the new mayor.[1]

It had been a long day for Newton and his fellow aldermen, and one heavily punctuated with eating and drinking. Newton lists what was put on the dinner table, and it appears from his account that these dishes came one after another, and presumably were served with sauces and bread which he does not mention. It is not clear whether the dishes were shared between diners, or whether, for instance, each diner received two boiled chickens.

On 21 October the university and the town usually met in Great St Mary's church for the Paving Leet, which fined those who had defaulted on paying the paving rate, and on 26 October the town court and leet, held in the Guildhall, included the Leet of Annoyances. When Newton was town treasurer he had to collect the fines ordered by these leets.[2]

The next occasion for civic feasting was following the sermon celebrating King James's deliverance from the Gunpowder Plot of 5 November. The dinner that followed the sermon consisted of two legs of veal and bacon, a large piece of roast beef, a loin and leg of pork, three couple of rabbits and two bottles of claret.[3] On 6 and 13 November the mayor and corporation attended the annual obit sermons for Alderman John Fan and Alderman Foxton who had left benefices to the town, including two booths at Stourbridge Fair, and money for the poor. Alderman Fan's obit sermon was followed by a 'collation of a sugar cake and one cup of sack for everyone present'.[4]

The plague meant that all of these functions were cancelled, and Samuel Newton and his fellow members of the corporation stayed at home. They went about their daily life as best they could, hoping that as the summer heat died down so the plague would abate, but quietly and insidiously it spread. Thomas Butt who lived in Holy Sepulchre parish (the Round Church) died of the plague on 29 September followed by his wife on 1 October 1665. The Butts left tiny orphans, and they too died, but whether this was of the plague is not known as they do not appear in the parish register; the Overseers of Poor's Account stated that the overseers of the poor 'Paid 2s to Dan for burying Butt's children' in October 1665. The overseers at this time were John Woods, Peter Dent and William

Witty, and this entry is evidence that Peter Dent stayed in Cambridge during the plague, and kept his apothecary's shop open.[5]

Holy Sepulchre was a small parish, with most of its houses clustered around its church and churchyard and at the town end of Bridge Street. Peter Dent's house abutted the churchyard; across the street from him Alderman Thomas Tifford lived 'west of the Sign of the Swan'. His neighbour, another alderman, John Ewin a chandler, had been mayor in 1660 and had had the honour of proclaiming the restoration of Charles II. Mr William Pedder, a gentleman, lived in a large house next to the walls of Sidney Sussex College. This house stood back from the street and had a front garden. In 1657 Pedder had illegally and without the corporation's planning permission erected a post and rail fence in front of his houses, and despite inspections by various aldermen, and orders to remove, refused to do so.[6]

Life had to go on. John Linsey, a fishmonger who lived in St Clement's but traded from a stall under the Purgold in Pease Hill,[7] continued to sell fish to his customers; freshwater carp, perch and pike were especially popular in the 1660s. He got these from the river or from the fish ponds in St Peter's parish. Barrels of oysters came from Brightlingsea in Essex, eels from the Fens were brought in by the licensed eel catchers, herrings soaked in brine or smoked 'red herrings' came down the river by barge from King's Lynn, as did the casks of sturgeon, favourites of the Cambridge aldermen. Anchovies, salmon and lobster were also fashionable dishes in seventeenth-century Cambridge.[8]

Fish could so easily rot, and during the hot summer of 1665 being a fishmonger was a chancy business. John Linsey survived the summer, but when his 14-year-old son Christopher, the fifth of his seven children, fell ill on 1 October he was worried. Christopher had been a delicate child, subject to the shivering fits and high temperatures which went with fen ague. Poppy juice was administered to him as a cure for the ague, but this was something much more serious. He died of the plague on 4 October, Linsey's house on Bridge Street was closed up, and his stall on the Purgold stood empty.[9] This gave Linsey's former apprentice Peter Lightfoot, who had been freed from his apprenticeship in 1656, a chance to capitalise on Linsey's misfortune and make an even better living. The Lightfoots were a family of fishmongers. Patrick Lightfoot was inspector of fish at Stourbridge Fair in 1660 and 1667, and Richard Lightfoot was inspector in 1664. Like John Linsey, Peter Lightfoot lived in St Clement's parish but sold his fish in the Market Place.[10]

It is with the next two plague victims in Holy Sepulchre that we get the first evidence of plague travelling from household to household and through extended families. Annis White of the parish and her sister Mary Fossett were both buried as plague victims on 2 October 1665. Annis was the wife of William White, a cooper, and Mary was married to William Fossett. They lived in a rented house next door to the Butts, who had also died from the plague. The only other member of their families to succumb to the infection was William White's son, another William, who died on 19 October 1665.[11]

On the day that William White died, a fellow who had stayed on in Clare College sent a letter to another fellow who had fled:

Alderman Myrrell the brewer and one of his children died of plague last Monday, he hath four children dead of it. Clayton the barber in Petty Cury and one of his children died last Saturday of the sickness. It is nearly broken out by Christ's College (though they are all fled from the college on account of Mr Bunchley, their manciple dying of the plague) where Nicholson the smith and his wife and three children died within three days, his other children deadly sick in the house. But it rageth most in St Clements parish, where never a day passeth without one dead of the sickness. Poor Mr Brown, the old man that is one of the University musicians and Mr Sanders that sings the deep bass are shut up in Mr Saunders house in Green Street, whose child died last week suspected. Two houses at Barton are infected. At [Fen] Ditton [it] is broke out by the butcher, from where we have our meat, which made us hastily remove to Grantchester. Henry Glenton the carrier fled from town to Shelford, where he died two or three days later suspected. Royston is sadly in two or three places infected. The last of which is just in the middle of the town. The infection they say brought thither by a Cambridge man, whom they caught and shut him up, but he hath since made his escape.[12]

Francis Nicholson, the smith mentioned in the letter, lived close to Christ's College, and rented a garden in Fair Yard Lane so that he could grow his own herbs and vegetables. His wife and child died on 13 and 14 October respectively.[13]

The Cambridge Bills of Mortality always start with the phrase 'All Colleges, (God Be Praised) are found to have continued without any infection of plague', but Mr Bunchley's death was evidence to the contrary. William Bunchley lived close to Christ's College in St Andrew's parish. As manciple he was in charge of purchasing goods for the college and issuing contracts. He had married Elizabeth Taylor of St Peter's parish in St Peter's church on 13 May 1636, and baptised three children in St Andrew's church, Elizabeth in 1639, William in 1643, Mary in 1646; the baptism of another child, Edward, has not been traced. (This may have taken place in Elizabeth's home parish of St Peter's and he was probably the eldest son.) Bunchley made his will early in 1665 while he was still healthy, and was buried as a plague victim on 4 October 1665. In his will he left £5 to his son Edward to buy a mourning gown, to his daughter

Elizabeth a house and pastures in Stow cum Quy, and to his daughter Mary £150. The rest of the household stuff was to be divided equally between them. The inventory of his house and possessions was not made until February 1668, when the appraisers could be sure that the last vestiges of plague had disappeared from them. Goods worth £249 18s. 11d were found in the parlour, fore chamber, second fore chamber, the Great Chamber over the parlour, and the kitchen. Bunchley's house had five hearths, so every room had a source of heat.[14]

The 'Alderman Myrrell' mentioned in the letter was Alderman Thomas Merriall who in 1665 shared a large house with the brewer Roger Thompson, while his own house was being renovated. As well as being a brewer Merriall had been inspector of hogs at Stourbridge Fair in 1656, and town treasurer in 1660. The Clare letter suggests he had at least five children, but only three of these can be traced, and they were still in St Clement's in September 1665, where Susanna who died of a 'spotted fever' was buried on 6 September and her sister Elizabeth on the 28th. Was this a cover-up and did the girls really die of the plague? If plague was seen as the sickness of the poor an alderman with a position to maintain would not want to be in the same situation as them. Neither he nor Roger Thompson would have wanted their house put into quarantine, but Thompson was aware that both girls could be suspected of dying from the plague, and prudently moved out to Chesterford in Essex, where he met his future wife.[15] If Elizabeth Merriall died of plague on 28 September, symptoms of which would include spots and a fever, a 12- to 14-day incubation period would account for the deaths of Thomas Merriall and his son Charles on 16 October: they are listed as plague victims in the parish register.[16]

Barton was a village about two miles south-west of Cambridge, with a population of some 130 in 1665. One family was hit by the plague; Mary, the daughter of Thomas Bonnet of Barton, was buried on 23 September, her sister Susan on the same day, their brother Thomas on 3 October and finally their father on 12 November 1665.[17]

The second week of October saw a flurry of plague deaths in St Clement's. The Nine Pins in Thompson's Lane was closed on 14 October when its landlord John Amey and his son, another John, died of the plague. There were three more burials on the same day that the Merrialls were buried, a further five on 19 October, one on the 25th and another on 30 October. Fifteen houses, inns and business were closed up, and the churchyard was getting full. Today St Clement's churchyard is raised about four feet above the road surface, due to continual use, and in 1665 there was some discussion as to whether the plague dead should be put into a communal grave or pit, as those who died in pest houses were, but there were objections to this. What would happen on the Day of Judgment? Would all those bodies jumbled together haphazardly in a pit be able to rise? Great pits were dug in London, where the dead lay 'piled up like faggots in a stack',[18] but the London plague pits were dug in unconsecrated ground, the bodies delivered at night in a cart and tipped into the pits without a burial service said over them. St Clement's parish did not want this, but it made compromises. Carts were used to collect the bodies rather than the parish bier; the body was sewn into the sheet in which the victim had died by grieving relatives, who then pushed the corpse into the street in response to the call of the bellman preceding the dead cart. There was no time to make coffins, as deaths came too thick and fast. The passing bell no longer tolled in Cambridge churches; instead the ministers said the burial service over the grave in the open air, alone apart from the gravediggers and the sexton. Mourners were forbidden to attend the service for fear of spreading the infection further.

In St Clement's parish, John Bird's house was still closed in October following the deaths of his daughters Ann and Jennet in August and September. John himself was taken to the pest house, where he too died. John's brother Nathaniel lived nearby on the west side of Bridge Street, next door to St John's College brew house.[19] The two families were in and out of each other's houses every day, so perhaps it was no surprise when Nathaniel's son Peter died of the plague on 7 October 1665, and despite his protests Nathaniel was taken to the pest house, where he died. His five-year-old son and his wife were buried on 16 October, leaving seven-year-old George Bird alone.[20]

A third Bird brother, Francis, was the landlord of the Ship Inn on the Quayside. This was a large inn and popular with travellers. It had twelve guest bedrooms, two parlours, one for the family and one for guests, three chambers, a hall and a kitchen, with a yard and stables for travellers' horses. In 1665 it was owned by John Hills, a baker, and leased to Francis Bird.[21] The inn needed a large staff to run it: a bevy of boys to hold and stable visitors' horses as well as ostlers and grooms, cooks and serving girls, chambermaids and porters.

When Francis Bird's wife Emm died in 1664 she left him with five small children to look after. Although his sisters-in-law helped when they could, he needed someone full-time to care for the children, so three months after Emm's death he married Ann Stamford. People might whisper and say that this was with undue haste, but most understood that Francis could not manage a large inn like the Ship and keep an eye on small children, especially when they kept escaping and playing dangerous games around the horses' hooves in the yard, or toddling too close to the river. When his son Thomas came down with signs of the plague, Francis was desperate. The inn would be closed, and how would they live? Thomas died on 12 November and his father five days later. The lease of the inn passed to Francis's widow Ann and his eldest daughter Elizabeth. Ann then married William Sell, a carter from Burwell who had been accustomed to stable his horses at the inn when in town, and they managed the inn between them. Elizabeth was the only one of Francis Bird's children to survive into adulthood.[22] By the end of November 1665 the Bird family had lost nine members, including the three family breadwinners.

Another large and extended family living in St Clement's were the Bullins. John Bullin the elder was a hatter and haberdasher. He lived and worked in Bridge Street, but also rented two tenements in Harleston's Lane from St John's College.[23]

Hats and hatbands were the predominant stock of the haberdasher, and by making the hats himself, John Bullin cut out the manufacturer. Haberdashers also stocked sewing materials, needles, thread, buckram for linings, silks, ribbons, tapes, buttons, pins and household items such as curtain rings and beeswax for polishing furniture.[24]

The hats John Bullin made were probably felt hats. Felt was made by compressing wool or rabbit fur with intense heat and moisture. Bullin's felt would have been rabbit fur from the nearby Breckland area of East Anglia, where part of the economy was based on rabbits.[25] A seventeenth-century woodcut of a hat-making workshop shows a back room where a man is heating and wetting fibres, and passing the congealed mass to three men in the front room who are seen rolling out the moisture from the fibres by hand, at a table with a drain underneath. Blocks for making the hat crowns lie on the floor. This suggests that John Bullin would have needed at least one or two assistants to make his hats. Continually working with heat, moisture and fibres must have led to industrial diseases such as emphysema.

Once the hats were made by John Bullin they were passed to his brother William, a hat dyer,[26] so there was evidently a Bullin production line of hats. William Bullin needed space for the dyeing process, and a ready supply of water. The dye was prepared in a cauldron over a source of heat and the article to be dyed was dipped in it for the required time; the dye was then set using a mordant of vitriol or copperas or, if the dye used was woad, the mordant was potash or argol, a substance scraped from the inside of a wine barrel. Woad, of course, produced a blue dye, madder from the roots of the *Rubia tinctoria* gave a red dye, weld, a yellow dye, could be obtained from the end of the branches of butcher's or dyer's broom, or could be obtained from saffron, which was grown locally in Cambridgeshire. Imported dyes such as indigo or orchil, which gave a purplish red, were much more expensive and rare, but could be obtained at Stourbridge Fair. Dark blues and blacks were produced by repeated dipping in woad and then adding madder to 'sadden' the colour. This was a time-consuming labour-intensive process, so a cheaper black dye was produced from oak galls, the excretion of larvae on oak trees, also known as oak apples.[27] This was probably the dye used by William Bullin for the ubiquitous black hats worn by men and women in seventeenth-century Cambridge. Once the dyeing was complete in one colour the residue from the cauldron had to be dumped. In William Bullin's case it was poured into the river.

A third Bullin brother, Adam, also lived in St Clement's, and in 1664 William Bullin the hat dyer moved into Adam's house with his son William, Joseph aged seven and a daughter, Eve.[28] Adam's daughter Sarah cared for William's younger children, and she became very fond of young Joseph. It was she who smuggled him treats from the kitchen, dried his tears when he fell down and told him stories at bedtime; and it was Sarah who noticed that Joseph was unwell and thought his runny nose might be more serious than an ordinary cold. Joseph died on 5 October, Sarah on 31 October, and her parents Adam and Sarah on 3 and 4 November.

The colder weather of November brought renewed hope that the plague would cease, but the plague burials continued, three more in St Clement's, one in St Andrew's parish, and Benjamin Trott in Holy Sepulchre parish. One of the foremost residents of Holy Sepulchre parish was Christopher Bumstead, an alderman and a brazier by trade, who lived in a large house with a workshop in the yard, next to the former mayor John Ewins.[29]

Christopher Bumstead was a skilled craftsman who worked with expensive materials: alloys of brass and latten and copper alloys. His workshop was equipped as a forge, with a hearth, bellows, melting pans, tongs, hammer, files, spindles and moulds. The metal was heated and poured into moulds made of stone, wood or metal, and then finished off by hammering and filing, while items such as candlesticks had the candle holders welded onto them. As well as candlesticks, Christopher Bumstead made chafing dishes, spice mortars, stirrups, buckles, copper bowls, pots and kettles. Nearly every household in Cambridge had at least one item from his workshop, and he could also make bespoke items decorated with enamel.[30] The noise of his hammering and the hiss of metal being cooled with water added to the street sounds, and in winter friends and neighbours liked to gather round the forge hearth and watch him at work.

Christopher and his wife Joan had nine children, ranging in age in 1665 from 25 to three years. Christopher, named for his father, was 13 in 1665, and was not yet apprenticed so still lived at home. When on 2 November he was taken with an incurable bout of the hiccoughs, his siblings found it extremely funny. His father tried to scare the hiccoughs out of him, his mother gave him a mug of water and told him to drink from the far side, his brothers tried tickling him, and one of his sisters dropped a cold knife down his back, but all to no avail: the hiccoughs went on and on. It was not until he collapsed with a thread of blood from his nose that his family realised that this

was more than mere indigestion.[31] He died of plague on 5 November
and his family were incarcerated in their home until 15 December.[32]

Without Christopher Bumstead's hammering ringing off the
walls of houses, the streets around Holy Sepulchre seemed eerily
silent. The sounds and smells of the town were changed by the
plague, and shut up in their houses Bumstead and other craftsmen
could not trade. They needed capital to buy raw materials: the Bullins
needed to buy dyestuffs and rabbit fur for their hats, Elias Woodward
the glazier needed capital to purchase sheets of glass, and John Linsey
had to buy his fish. There was no money coming in while they were
shut up in their houses, and money was going out for provisions. The
plague was an economic disaster for them.

December the 6th was declared a national fast day for the plague. It
seemed that with a cold spell the plague might abate, but the weather
changed to warm and muggy in the second week of the month, and
plague cases began to increase again.[33] On 10 December Richard
Cutchey's daughter Elizabeth died of the plague. Richard Cutchey
lived next door to the Ship in St Clement's. His one-storey hovel was
dwarfed by the three-storey inn.[34] Despite its small size Richard and
his wife managed to raise five children in their hovel, but with the close
proximity of the plague-ridden inn, it came as no surprise when
Richard's daughter Elizabeth died. There were now two buildings
closed on the Quayside, and Portugal Place off Bridge Street was closed
on 12 December when the son and daughter of John Bestoe died.[35]

The Cambridge Bills of Mortality for 30 November to 14
December list twelve burials, including four of plague and four more
admitted to the pest house; those for 14 December to 28 December
list twelve burials including seven of plague victims and another four
sent to the pest house. Twenty unnamed people from St Peter's
parish died in the pest house between October and December 1665.
The year drew to a sombre close. Between September and December

1665, 33 houses were shut up in St Clement's (35 per cent of all its property), and 56 houses were closed in the town as a whole, imprisoning about 250 men, women and children.[36]

Not everyone agreed with shutting up infected houses, and imprisoning the sick and the well inside, but order number 5 of the Privy Council's Plague Orders stated that 'The houses of those infected were to be closed for 5 weeks ...', and this had to be obeyed. The physician Nathaniel Hodges, who remained in London throughout the plague in 1665 and 1666, thought that shutting up infected houses added to the death toll and that 'the consternation of those shut up in the house with the victims was inexpressible'; while shutting up houses made neighbours fly who otherwise might help the stricken. In some houses where corpses lay awaiting burial, from:

> Persons in their last Agonies: in one Room might be heard dying Groans ... and not far off ... infants passed immediately from the Womb to the Grave ... the infected run about staggering like drunken Men, and fall and expire in the Streets; while others lie half-dead and comatose, but never to be waked but by the last Trumpet ...

Hodges acknowledged that shutting up houses was for the 'Publick Good', but suggested that 'if plague should break out again, the infected should be moved outside the city into purpose built apartments'.[37]

Hodges's contemporary, the apothecary William Boghurst thought that 'As soon as any house is infected, all the sound people should be had out of it, and not shut up therein and murdered.'[38] Dr Richard Kingston, the parson of Clerkenwell broke into verse to describe the stricken houses when he wrote to his churchwardens on 18 October 1665:

But with a sad 'Lord Have Mercy Upon Us', and
A bloody cross, as fatal marks did stand,
Presaging the noisome pestilence within
Was come to take revenge on us for sin.[39]

In Cambridge the Plague Orders decreed that every infected house should have two watchmen, one for day and one for night, each paid 8d a day,[40] a great strain on the town's finances. The Bumstead family who had seven children, the youngest only three years old, were shut up in their house from the beginning of November to mid-December, anxiously watching for signs of the plague to appear and relying on the goodwill of neighbours to leave food and drink outside the house for them. Elias Woodward, the glazier, and his wife were shut up in their house and watched four of their children die of the plague, and when Thomas and Katherine Butt died they left small children in the infected house, bewildered and frightened. Neighbours saw their little faces staring hopefully out of the windows, until they too died. When husbands such as Robert Leake of St Giles died, their widows were left to fend for themselves and their children.

On 22 December there was a hard frost.[41] Frost in Cambridge rimed the windows, hardened the ground and painted the trees white. Christmas approached and with it the hope of an infection-free 1666.

CHAPTER 7

A Rash of Red Crosses

FOR MANY PEOPLE in Cambridge, Christmas was a religious day. In normal times Samuel Newton took communion in his own church, St Edward's, in the morning, and joined a scarlet clad procession of aldermen to hear a sermon at Great St Mary's in the afternoon.[1] Isaac Archer a clergyman from Trinity College, Cambridge usually spent the day examining his conscience, while Samuel Pepys went to church to hear a sermon and then either went home or to an alehouse for cakes and ale. In the evening a wassail woman came to his house with a bowl of wassail ale, and sang carols for alms and a mug of ale, and in 1662 Pepys had 'a brave plum pudding, a roasted pullet and mince pies', although his wife did not make her 'Christmas Pies', until 26 December.[2]

Before they were suppressed during the Commonwealth and rule of Oliver Cromwell, Christmas had been a day for revels and games, and churches were decorated with greenery. There were riots against the Puritan Christmas at Bury St Edmunds, Norwich and Ipswich, but not at Cambridge, and Newton's diary suggests that for the middle rank of society which he belonged to New Year's Day and the two days following were the days for feasting and meeting neighbours.[3]

However, in the five years between the Restoration of Charles II and the onset of the plague the church bells would have rung out across the town on Christmas Eve, and the town and university waits serenaded the birth of Christ. Mummers would have performed their plays in the streets, in the courtyards of inns and colleges, and visited larger houses in the town, and the Molly dancers, young men dressed up as women, pranced in from the surrounding Fens in search of largesse. Christmas was a time for giving alms and distributing doles.

Few in Cambridge ventured out to church on 25 December 1665. Instead the population stayed quietly in their houses and the festivities were muted. The mayor's feast for the town's sergeants, gaolers and their wives was cancelled, and so was his feast for the aldermen.[4]

One family that stayed indoors over Christmas were the Kelseys. The head of the family was William Kelsey, a baker who lived in St Giles parish in premises leased from Clare College, and next door to Artemus Hinde the apothecary. They had moved there from Holy Sepulchre parish across the river, and they had a son and two grown-up daughters. Elizabeth was married to Robert Bartholomew and they had presented William with a grandson named after him, who was three at Christmas 1665. They lived across the river in Holy Sepulchre parish. Kelsey's other daughter, Edith, was married to James Wendy who was apprenticed to his father Thomas, a butcher of St Clement's. Usually, the families got together in the family home in St Giles, but this year they decided it was safer to stay in their own houses; however, William baked Christmas loaves with honey and raisins and sent them to his daughters, then spent the day in front of his fire. His wife roasted a couple of rabbits on a spit, and they drank Christmas ale warmed with a hot poker. But William, who was a devout and religious man, missed going to church. In his will, drawn up in July 1667, he described himself as the 'unprofitable servant of God'. He left his business to his son provided he maintained his mother in 'a good, wholesome and sufficient manner with meat and apparel and other things needful for the term of her natural life, without collusion or rowing'. She was to be paid 30s. a year, and he left bequests to his sons-in-law and daughters. He asked to be buried in St Giles church, and he got his wish: he was buried there in February 1668.[5] All the Kelseys survived the plague, and William the younger continued the bakery business in St Giles.

On Christmas Day 1665 in London, Samuel Pepys ventured out to his parish church and to his amazement saw a wedding, 'which I had not seen for many a day, young people so merry one with each other'.[6] Life could go on despite the plague, and people in Cambridge looked forward to the New Year with some optimism.

Samuel Newton celebrated his seventh wedding anniversary in January; his wife Sarah was pregnant with their second son. The university should have reopened at the beginning of January 1666, but on the 23rd Dr Francis Wilford, the university vice-chancellor wrote to its chancellor the Earl of Manchester asking him to obtain a letter from the king empowering the university to choose the time when they reconvened, as 'they dare not call home their company, by reason of the sickness'. On 19 February the king gave them permission to delay the reopening until the first Sunday in Lent. He added that the same could be done in any year the plague threatened, thus removing the necessity for frequent royal letters.[7]

The Cambridge parish registers state that there were five plague deaths between January and February 1666; however, although the Bills of Mortality record that in the week from 28 December 1665 to 4 January 1666 the town was clear of the plague, the next week the Bills record four plague deaths, two in Barnwell on the outskirts of the town, and two in St Clement's. The following week there were three plague burials, one in Barnwell and two in St Clement's, and the week after one death in the pest house, but this was not from plague.[8] Mary Chappell of St Clement's died of plague on 5 January, as did Ann Griggs, daughter of Moses Griggs, landlord of the Crow on Bridge Street. Jeremiah Brewer and Ann Gray perished from the plague on 16 January, and Ann Woodward, the daughter of Felix Woodward a fisherman, on 28 January. Hers was the last plague death in St Clement's in that winter of 1666. The next deaths recorded in the parish register were from 'rising of the lights' (Susanna Crosby), 'a stopping' (Esther Wingfield), and three deaths from consumption, those of Widow Elizabeth Lamb, of Elinor daughter of Thomas Morgan, and of Thomas son of Thomas Brigham.[9]

By March it looked as if optimism had been rewarded and Cambridge was clear of plague, and an announcement to that effect was placed in the *London Gazette* of 19–22 March 1666: 'This place is now (God be praised) free from infection, not one having died here these six weeks, so that all that return hither will be received and we hope without danger: upon which confidence the first Act for B. As [Bachelors of Arts] is appointed for 2nd April, and the latter 26th April.'[10]

College rooms were aired. Dons packed their books and returned from the country, and young men flocked into town with their luggage. College bells pealed again, and the sound of young voices was heard once more in college corridors. The market reopened and farmers began to bring produce into town. The cook shops relit their fires, and music from the town and university waits permeated the streets. The town and university breathed a collective sigh of relief: surely the worst was over, and they had survived.

One of the dons who returned to Cambridge was Henry More of Christ's College who had spent the duration of the summer plague at Ragley Hall in Warwickshire with Lady Anne Conway. Anne had been introduced to More by her brother John Finch while he was a scholar at Christ's College, and a friendship and long-term correspondence started between More and Lady Conway. John Finch had all the advantages of a university education and a Grand Tour of Europe, while Anne, who was obviously an intelligent woman, received neither of these. Despite this, More wrote to her as an intellectual equal, and his letters were a welcome distraction when her husband was absent on his Irish estates. One of their mutual interests was their health. Both More and Lady Conway suffered from debilitating headaches, which they delighted in comparing. Lady Conway was desperate for a cure, and she wrote to More asking for his opinion of Matthew Croker, a faith healer who claimed to be able to cure by merely speaking to a sufferer. More was sceptical about Croker, being more inclined to believe in the powers of Valentine Greatrakes, who induced cures by 'stroking'.[11]

Valentine Greatrakes claimed to be able to cure the plague as well as other ailments, and it was Lady Conway's husband who 'discovered' him at Youghall [sic] in Ireland in July 1665. Greatrakes came from a gentry family who had supported Cromwell but had escaped punishment at the Restoration, and had retired to their Irish estates. In 1661 Greatrakes claimed to have had a sudden impulse that he could touch and heal for the King's Evil (scrofula), and that the gift was bestowed on him by God.[12] This claim was dangerous, as only an anointed king could touch for the King's Evil, but his fame spread, and the sick flocked to him; it was then that he was discovered by Lord Conway.

Conway, perhaps tired of his wife's headaches, immediately transported him to Ragley Hall where Lady Conway and Henry More were in residence. Before treating Lady Conway it was decided that Greatrakes should try out his cure on Conway's tenants. The sick or lame tenants on the estate, and servants in the house, were rounded up and stroked by Greatrakes, and then examined by Henry More, who pronounced them cured. The stage was set to try out the cure on Lady Conway. Greatrakes laid his hands on her head. Nothing happened. She was no better, and the headaches continued. [13]

Greatrakes left Ragley Hall and went to London where he was besieged by people wanting a cure for the plague. Of course, he could not cure the plague, and when he failed to cure Sir John Denham, who subsequently went 'stark mad', he prudently withdrew to Ireland.[14] He was one of the many tricksters who preyed on people's fear of the plague and forlorn hope that a cure could be found.

March was dry and cold, and at the end of the month there were drought conditions, but on 3 April there were some small showers, 'very refreshing to our dusty land'. Showers continued through April, and the climate was 'warm and close'.[15] The warm, damp spring meant that crops were growing well in the fields, and there would be a good harvest.

Despite Cambridge's relief that the plague had ceased, the town's optimism received a blow on 25 May 1666 when Midsummer Fair was cancelled by royal proclamation, 'for fear of spreading infection to Cambridge, which is now free'.[16] The town was disappointed, but perhaps it was better to keep strangers away and keep the town healthy, and on 29 May the king's birthday was celebrated with church bells pealing all day.

There had been an interlude in the Dutch War in the autumn and winter of 1665–66, but in January France and Denmark joined Holland and declared war on England. Charles retaliated by declaring war on them on 11 February 1666, but the fleet did not put to sea until early May.[17] The Dutch and English fleets engaged off Ostend on 1 June, in what became known as the Four Days' Battle. The English fleet was forced to withdraw to Sheerness miserably shattered and mangled and with a hardly a vessel entire.[18] Another engagement, off the Dutch island of Terschelling, resulted in the English sinking 150 Dutch merchant ships; it was hailed as a great victory, and the church bells rang out once again. But public morale was sapped by the plague, and there was no stomach for the war. Pressed men were desperately needed to man the fleet, but because only towns free from the plague were plundered for men, discontent against press gangs was growing. A report to the government from its commissioner in King's Lynn said he had managed to impress seventy able-bodied seamen with the assistance of shipmasters. Lynn itself was still healthy, and a 'watch was kept to prevent people from Cambridge, Norwich and Peterborough where the sickness is from coming in'.[19]

It started in the parish of St Botolph where travellers from London entered the town. In 1665 they had to show a certificate of health, but this procedure was relaxed when the town was declared free of plague in March 1666.

St Botolph's huddled around Trumpington Street and the lanes leading off it. In the sixteenth century most of the cottages had back-yards, but by the seventeenth century most of these were in-filled; however, Bow Green was still an open space, with grass and trees. Penny Farthing Lane, which lay beside St Botolph's churchyard, had one row of houses in the sixteenth century, but by the seventeenth century this was a double row, back to back across what had once been a yard.[20]

The Ellingworth sisters Jane and Ann lived with their father in a cottage on Penny Farthing Lane. They had moved to Cambridge in 1664, and survived the infection of 1665.[21] Jane was a seamstress working from their cottage's front room, and Ann was a college laundress, while their father was a part-time general labourer, and full-time tippler, which was why they had moved to Cambridge: the girls had to find work. Their income had been curtailed during the plague months of 1665 so that they were forced to ask the parish for relief, and they received altogether £1 8s. 6d.[22] On Wednesday 6 June, Ann went to her work as usual, but Jane sat listless with her sewing untouched in her lap. Despite his lapses from sobriety Thomas loved his daughters and he brought Jane a cup of small ale and persuaded her to lie on her bed. She died the next day, the first victim of the 1666 plague in Cambridge, and Ann died on 16 June. Thomas survived, perhaps too pickled to succumb to the infection, but when on 26 July he stumbled out blinking into the sunshine he found the town's trade at a standstill, and there was no work available. He applied for poor relief and received 4s. 1d to tide him over.[23]

The plague had returned to Cambridge, and its townsmen would play no further part in the Dutch War. The young men and the dons packed up their belongings again and departed. College gates slammed shut and were locked. Traders stopped coming into town, and one by one the red crosses reappeared on the doors of houses.

For the time being, however, the plague had finished with St Botolph's parish, where now only two houses were shut up. But the infection was gathering pace elsewhere. Between 12 and 22 June there were thirteen plague deaths in St Andrew's parish. The infection started in the Hignell household, when an unnamed child of John Hignell was diagnosed as having died of the plague on 12 June, followed by John Hignell's wife on the 18th. In the Pate household Margery, John Pate's wife died on 14 June, and their near neighbour John Squire lost his daughter Mary aged 13 on 19 June.[24] Another St Andrew's resident was John Squire, a carpenter, who leased a piece of waste ground near where he lived. Here he built a shed to store his tools and wood, where he could escape from everyday life. Soon his house was also painted with a foot-high red cross 'evident to be seen' in the middle of the front door.[25]

The row of houses where the Hignells, Pates and Squires lived was to suffer more plague deaths. Next door to John Pate lived Nicholas Booth and his family. He was a say weaver: say was one of the new draperies, a fine woollen worsted fabric with silk added to it, which was used for luxury items such as tablecloths, bed covers, wall hangings and curtains. It was an expensive fabric, available only to the wealthier members of society. The green say curtains that appeared in William Bunchley's 1665 inventory had likely been purchased from Nicholas Booth. Nicholas had probably learned his trade in Colchester, the centre of say weaving, before he moved to Cambridge where he perceived a gap in the market. He was in Cambridge by 1640 when his daughter Hannah was baptised in St Andrew the Great parish church, followed by Marie in 1642, John in 1645, and Grace in 1652. An elder sister Sarah had been baptised before Nicholas moved to Cambridge.[26]

Production of the fabric involved the whole family, who lived and worked with their father. Katharine their mother and Grace sorted and combed the wool with teasels mounted on wooden handles, while Hannah and Marie spun it into yarn, and Sarah kept the books and served in the shop. John had his own loom like his father's. Grace and her mother had the worst job. They had to remove twigs, thorns and dung from the wool before they could comb and straighten it, but as they worked the women sang softly in harmony to the rhythm of Hannah and Marie's spinning wheels. The wool they were working with in June 1666 was especially scratchy and Grace and her mother complained about the fleabites they got from it. Nicholas had purchased the wool from Norwich, a known plague hot-spot, so when his wife and Grace fell ill he was very worried, and when the searchers arrived and declared they had the plague, he could not forgive himself. His wife died on 28 June 1666 and Grace the day after. Nicholas sewed their bodies into lengths of fine cloth, and when he heard the bellman announcing the arrival of the dead cart it was he who hollered 'Here!' and pushed their bodies through the door to be taken away. He had done his best for them.

When his wife fell ill, Nicholas, always a prudent man, made his will in case he too should be taken by the infection. It stated that he was in perfect health and sound memory, 'praise be to God'. He bequeathed his soul into the hands of God who had given it and left his son John and daughters Sarah, Hannah, Marie and Grace his household goods to be divided equally between them, or between those who survived. He asked that John be given 40s. immediately after his demise, and he named John and Sarah as his executors. Probate was granted on 22 March 1667.[27]

Nicholas was mistaken to think that he had brought the infection into his house with wool purchased in Norwich, as yet another household in his row of houses was stricken with the plague. The Tippings lived two doors away from the Pates and three from Nicholas Booth, so this was probably a case of infected rats with their infective blocked fleas moving from house to house. John Tipping died on 29 June, and was followed to the grave by his son, baby daughter and wife Frances.[28]

The rash of red crosses continued in St Andrew's parish. Charles Andrew's son died on 20 June, as did William Stubbins and Ann Fenn. They came from the poorer end of the parish where the houses were much smaller than those where the Pates, Booths and Squires lived.[29] On the same day John Bowles aged 26 from Holy Trinity parish died of the plague. His mother was William Stubbins's sister, and he might have received the fatal fleabite while visiting his uncle. The Bowles were too poor to pay the Hearth Tax; Alexander the father made a precarious living hawking beer round the streets in jugs and in 1655 had been fined for selling beer from illegal unmeasured jugs at Stourbridge Fair.[30]

Charles and Mary Andrews had married on 23 September 1662 and their children had come thick and fast, so that their tiny one-up, one-down cottage in Walls Lane (now King Street) was awash with toddlers: little Charlie, born a few months after their marriage, the twins Thomas and Mary baptised in June 1664, and baby Richard born in April 1666. They might be poor, but Charles was a good man who tried to provide for his family. He loved looking down at the sea of little heads thronging round him and loved to stroke their soft brown hair and listen to their childish prattle. He was distraught when Charlie died, followed by Thomas. The Andrews were shut into the house with their remaining children, but they were lucky in their neighbours, as widow Jane Mascall waited until the watch set outside the house was otherwise engaged, and smuggled in milk for the children and bread to sop in it.[31]

On Saturday 23 June 1666 Samuel Newton left his little enclave in plague-free St Edward's parish and moved his family to Waterbeach, five miles north-east of Cambridge on the west bank of the River Cam.[32] Here the Fens are extremely flat, and well below sea level. There was a ferry across the Cam at Clay Hythe, and in the village the ruins of Denny Abbey; about 120 houses clustered round the village green, with scattered farmsteads out on the Fens. The village had a population of about 500 when Newton moved there. Its economy was based on grazing sheep and cattle on the Fens, and growing wheat and barley where arable farming was possible.

Newton does not mention where he stayed in Waterbeach or with whom, but possibly it was either with John Knight, gentleman, or Anne Knight, widow, both of whom lived in substantial houses. Newton's sister Deborah was married to an Andrew Knight of London, who may have originated in Cambridgeshire.[33]

What did Newton do in his self-imposed exile? His clerks could have brought work out to him, but contact with them would have defeated the object of moving away from the threat of infection. Perhaps he enjoyed conversation with John Knight and others of a similar social standing in the village; the vicar, for example, or John and Jeremy Robson described as gentlemen who might have welcomed him into their houses. He probably took books and papers with him when he moved out of town, and may have taken musical instruments to entertain himself and for his son to practise on. Perhaps he took up fishing and spent long lazy summer afternoons sitting by the Cam with a rod in his hand and a hat over his eyes. This seems unlikely. Newton was a thoroughly urban man who enjoyed civic life, and he must have chafed at the inaction forced on him by his decision to move to the countryside. Plague did not follow him to Waterbeach, and there are no unusual burial patterns in the Waterbeach parish register.[34] But in the neighbouring parish of Landbeach across the Fens there were plague deaths, which gave rise to an enduring tale: 'According to legend, two old ladies ran away from the plague in London and came to Landbeach, to the house since called the Plague House, only for it to become apparent that they had brought it with them.' The legend reports that no one in the village died apart from the rector's son and servants; the rector's 'handwriting over the next few months suggests that he was shattered by the happenings and sank, a broken man, steadily through his final year and a half'.[35] Jack Ravensdale, who wrote this, took his story from W.K. Clay's *A History of the Parish of Landbeach*.[36]

Plague is not mentioned as a cause of death in the Landbeach burial register, but that does contain the germ of the legend. In 1666 there were sixteen burials between June and August, compared with the usual two, which suggests an epidemic. The dead included William Mead, a stranger, on 9 June 1666, and the 'two old ladies' Mrs Amy Brightmer, daughter of John Brightmer of Norwich, who died on 23 July, and Margaret, wife of Richard Potto, who died on

6 August. They were probably already infected when they reached Landbeach, as Norwich was badly hit by the plague by that time, and Margaret Potto was related to John, Obadiah and Dorothy Lord who all died of the plague in Cambridge on 18, 19 and 21 July 1666 respectively.[37] They may have been incarcerated in what is now known as 'The Plague House'.

The *Victoria County History ... Cambridgeshire* repeats the story that the refugees came from London. The legend that the rector's sorrow for the death of his son was reflected in his handwriting in the parish register is sentimental and inaccurate supposition. Landbeach is one parish where we know that the parish clerk wrote the registers, because in 1639 a special rate was levied in the parish for the clerk's wages, and this included among his duties the registration of marriages, baptisms and burials.[38]

On 24 June 1666 Lancelot, the son of Lancelot Hooper and his wife Christian of St Andrew's parish, died of the plague. Lancelot senior was a heel-maker, making wooden heels for shoes and boots. This brought a modest living, which Christian eked out by selling beer. In 1666 they had five children aged under ten, and living with them was William Thatcher, a parish apprentice taken on by Lancelot from St Edward's parish.[39] Lancelot Hooper was a Dissenter, whose house was licensed as a Congregationalist meeting place, but he had to baptise and bury his children in the parish church from necessity.[40]

Hooper was an affable man, who was on good terms with the minister, clerk and sexton of the parish church. They all enjoyed a good argument over a mug of ale, debating religious issues and commenting on the affairs of the day. Hooper asked the minister: was it the wickedness of mankind, and especially the debauchery of the court, that had brought the plague upon them? The euphoria of the Restoration had evaporated. Charles had been revealed as a

shallow, amoral man, and decent people gasped at his many bejew-
elled mistresses dressed in silk and satin, driving around London in
sumptuous carriages, while the sailors who manned the ships that
defended the country against the Dutch went unpaid, and their
families starved. Decent people hated the sight of Charles's mistresses
and their bastards flaunting themselves, while his wife, the little
Portuguese Catherine of Braganza, was neglected and childless. True,
she was a Catholic, but she deserved better.

Townspeople from Cambridge had only to travel a few miles to
the races at Newmarket to see the dazzling but debauched court for
themselves. It was fun to wave at the coaches and ask 'Who was
that?' but not for long. The splendour of the court was at odds with
the poverty they saw in the streets of Cambridge and the villages
surrounding Newmarket.

Lancelot Hooper lived to be a very old man, dying in 1701. His
inventory shows that he lived in a five-roomed house. Downstairs
were a kitchen, hall and parlour, and upstairs were the hall and
parlour chambers. Most of his possessions were described as very old
and had probably been purchased fifty years earlier when he was first
married. In his old age he slept in a four-poster bed in the hall
chamber, and kept his belongings in an old hanging press, a chest of
drawers, two trunks and a chest. The room contained a large amount
of linen, four chairs, a fire-brass, a looking glass, two silver spoons
and a brandy taster, as well as a parcel of old hangings. There were
two more beds in the parlour chamber, as well as a table and six
chairs. The kitchen contained cooking utensils and a large amount of
pewter – 28 dishes, 21 plates and 18 pots – while the hall, which
would have been the main living space, held two old tables, six chairs
and four stools, with a further 12 chairs in the parlour.[41] The pewter
and the large number of chairs were connected to Hooper's role as
host for Congregationalist meetings.

The Cambridge Bills of Mortality for 26 June to 3 July list 31 burials, of which 25 are of plague victims, with a further 11 people in the pest houses. St Andrew the Great was the epicentre of the plague at this time, and the King's Ditch went through this parish. In summer it was pungent with rubbish and effluvia, and this summer dead and dying rats lay along its banks. As the plague intensified the churchwardens decided to do something about the ditch for, as everybody knew, the plague was spread by bad air and smell. Four shillings were spent on scouring the section of ditch in St Andrew's. John How and his neighbour were part of the team of labourers who dug out the ditch and cleared the dead rats; John How and his child died of the plague on 22 June 1666.[42]

As well as in St Andrew's parish, red crosses could be seen in Holy Trinity, St Bene't's and St Botolph's. As the plague tightened its grip on Cambridge in June 1666, many looked at their world and wondered where it would end.

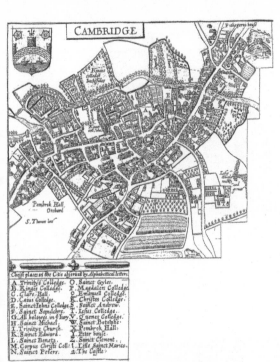

1. John Speed's Map of Cambridge 1610, taken from the *Theatre of the Empire of Great Britain*. It shows that the central plan of the town is similar to that of today.

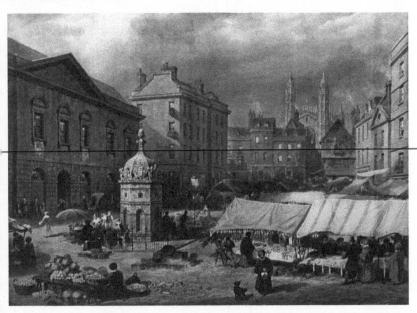

2. Cambridge Market Place with Hobson's Conduit. The conduit, which contained fresh water from Trumpington Nine Wells was given to the town by Thomas Hobson in 1614.

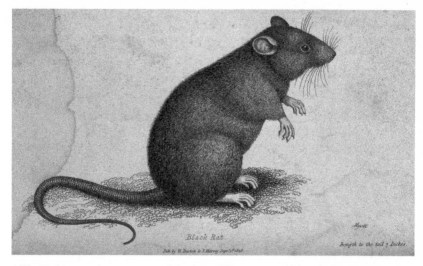

3. The black rat was the main vector of the plague. When it succumbed to the disease, its fleas then carried the infection across to humans.

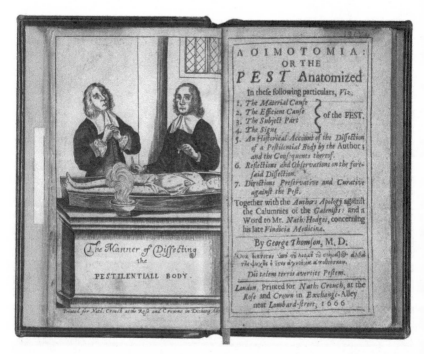

4. This shows George Thomson a physician dissecting the body of a fifteen-year-old plague victim, helped by his servant. Sulphur is burnt next to the victim to prevent the infection of the dissectors.

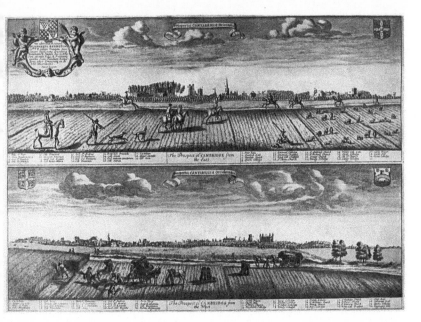

5. View of Cambridge from the East and the West by David Loggan. The spires of King's College chapel are in the distance.

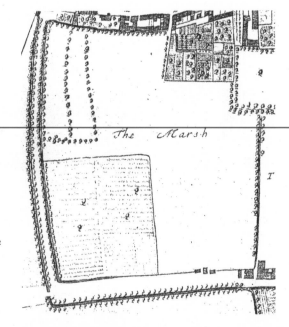

6. Willows fringing Cambridge roads, extract from David Loggan's Map of Cambridge, 1688. Willows were a cash crop in seventeenth-century Cambridge, and were planted whereever it was possible.

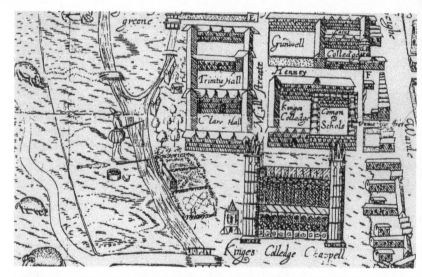

7. Fishing in the River Cam, extract from Richard Lyne's Map of Cambridge, 1574. The Cam was used for leisure as well as by women for washing clothes. But, polluted by nuisances, and domestic and industrial discharges, it was not used for drinking water.

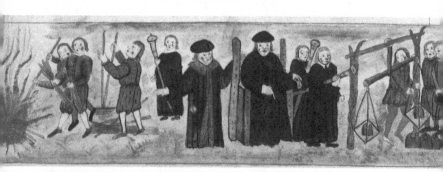

8. The vice-chancellor of Cambridge University inspects weights and measures in the market. Control of the town's weights and measures was one of the university's privileges. The vice-chancellor is accompanied by three bedells with maces.

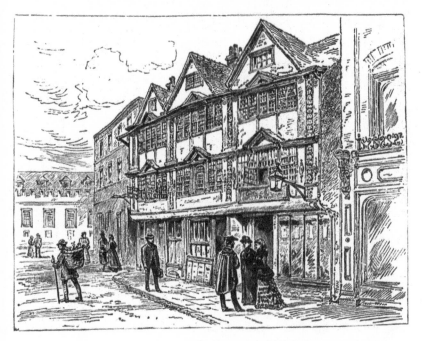

9. Double-fronted half-timbered houses in Trinity Street, from W.H. Redfern, *Old Cambridge*, 1876. The occupants of these houses, which were built in about 1600, would have experienced successive outbreaks of plague in the seventeenth century.

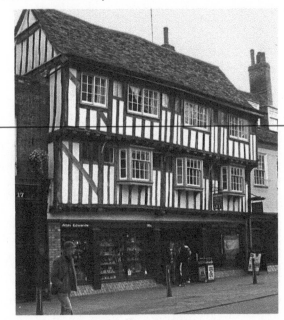

10. Half-timbered house in Bridge Street. Bridge Street was the main entry into the town from the north. In the seventeenth century this building would have been one of the many inns lining the street.

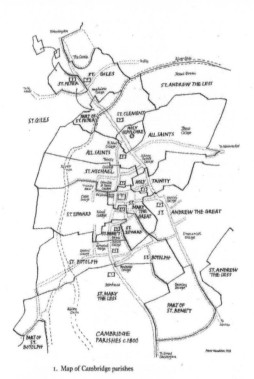

11. Map of Cambridge Parishes. The map shows that some parishes crossed the river and others, such as St Bene'ts, had detached portions away from the parish church.

1. Map of Cambridge parishes

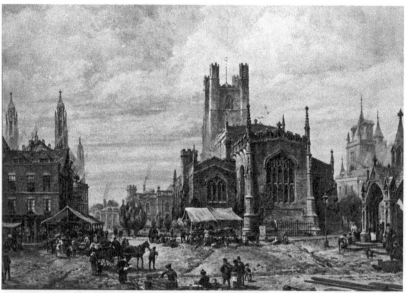

12. Great St Mary's Church and the Market Place. Great St Mary's was the most important parish church in the town, shared by the university and the corporation.

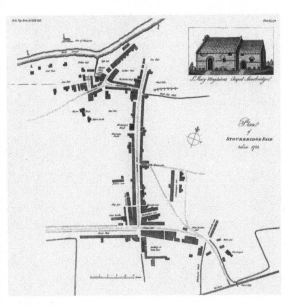

13. Plan of Stourbridge Fair Site, from J. Nichols, *The History and Antiquities of Barnwell Abbey and of Stourbridge Fair*, 1786. This shows the permanent layout of streets on the fair site, where timber booths were erected during the fair.

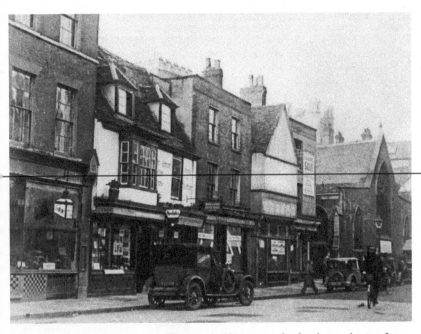

14. St Edward's Church from the east. The white building next to the church is on the site of Alderman Samuel Newton's house.

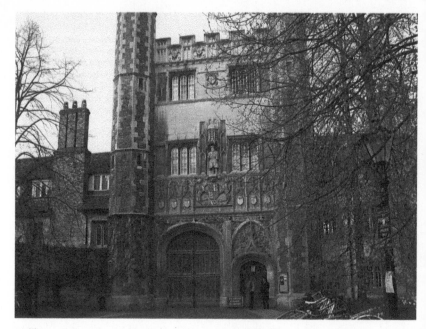

15. Trinity College, Cambridge. Sir Isaac Newton entered Trinity as a sizar in 1660.

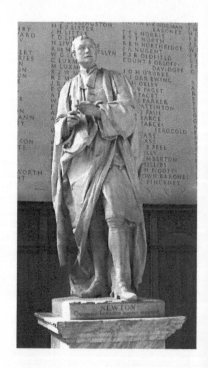

16. Sir Isaac Newton. During the great plague of 1665–6 Sir Isaac left Cambridge and returned home to Lincolnshire.

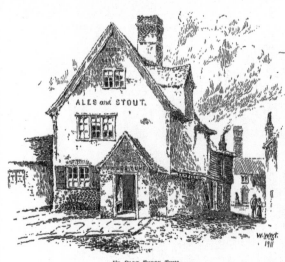

YE OLDE THREE TUNS.

17. *The Three Tuns*, drawing by W. West made in 1911 and published in A. Gray, *Cambridge Revisited*, based on newspaper articles in 1912. The Three Tuns was in St Edward's parish. In 1660 on a visit to Cambridge Samuel Pepys 'drank pretty hard' there.

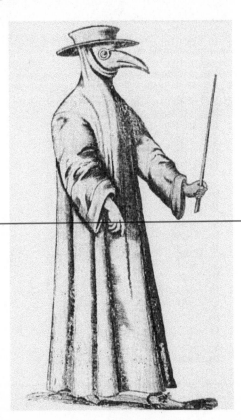

18. The Plague Doctor. The doctor wears a mask of oiled cloth with beak filled with aromats, and carries a white stave to show he is on the way to see a plague victim.

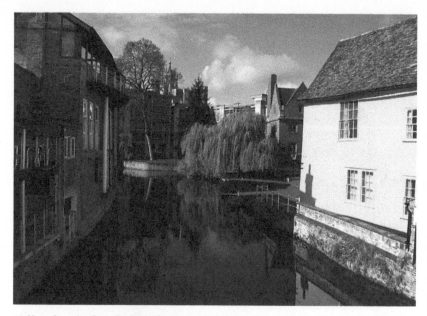

19. View from the Great Bridge looking towards St John's College. This is where the St Clements teenagers gathered in the summer of 1665.

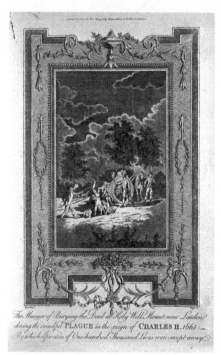

The Manner of Burying the Dead at Holy Well Mount near London during the dreadful PLAGUE in the reign of CHARLES II. 1665. By which if sways of One hundred Thousand Lives were swept away.

20. Burying the Dead in 1665. The dead are being thrown into a plague pit by moonlight.

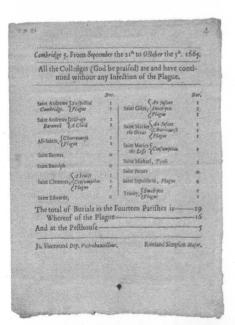

21. Cambridge Bills of Mortality,
21 September to 5 October 1665.
Cambridge issued fortnightly Bills of
Mortality in 1665, but as the plague
worsened these appeared weekly.

Cambridge 5. From September the 21ᵗʰ to October the 5ᵗʰ. 1665.

All the Colledges (God be praised) are and have continued without any Infection of the Plague.

	Bur.		Bur.
Saint Andrews {Suspected	1	Saint Giles, {An Infant	1
Cambridge. {Plague	1	{Small-pox	1
		{Plague	1
Saint Andrews {Old-age	1		
Barnwell {A Child	1	Saint Maries {An Infant	1
		the Great {Over-worn	1
All-Saints, {Clear-convst	1	{Plague	1
{Plague	1		
		Saint Maries {Consumption	1
Saint Bennet	0	the Lese	
Saint Botolph	0	Saint Michael, Teeth	1
		Saint Peters	0
Saint Clements {A bruise	1		
{Consumption	1	Saint Sepulchres, Plague	4
{Plague	7		
		Trinity, {Small-pox	1
Saint Edwards,	0	{Plague	1

The total of Burials in the Fourteen Parishes is————29
        Whereof of the Plague————————16
And at the Pesthouse————————————5

Ja. Fleetwood *Dep. Vice-chancellour.*   Rowland Simpson *Major.*

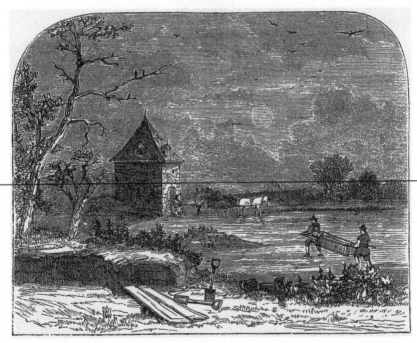

22. Pest House and Plague Pits in Finsbury Fields, London. One pest house is shown here but
there were clusters of these wooden huts on commons in Cambridge.

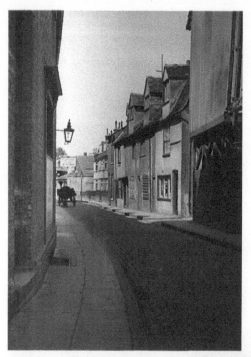

23. Thompson's Lane, St Clements Parish. Thompson's Lane was the home of many plague victims, including Alderman Merriall and his son.

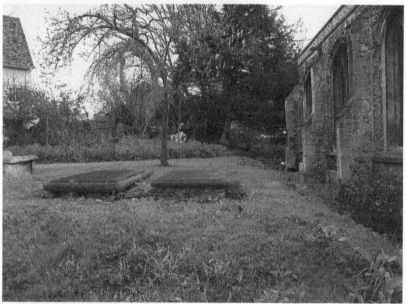

24. St Clements Graveyard. Today the graveyard is raised four feet above the road due to the tiers of bodies underneath the grass.

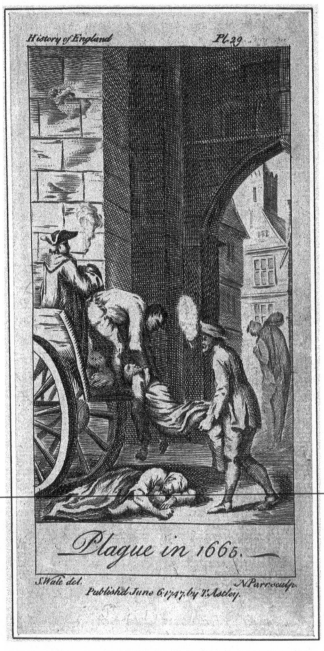

S.Wale del.   N.Parr sculp.

Publish'd June 6 1747. by T.Astley.

25. Plague victims being bundled out of a house. This dramatic interpretation
shows the victims wrapped in the sheets in which they died, and the carriers
smoking pipes to ward off infection.

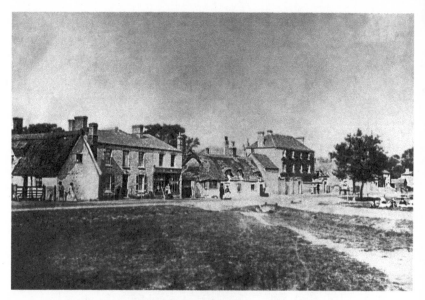

26. Waterbeach Village Green. In the summer of 1666 Alderman Samuel Newton and his family moved to Waterbeach to escape the plague in Cambridge.

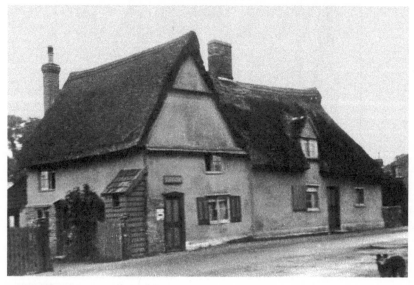

27. The Plague House, Landbeach. Traditionally, this is where the village's plague victims were housed. They had fled from plague spots, bringing the infection with them.

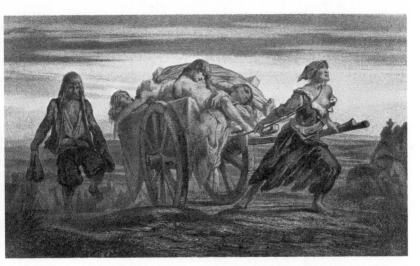

28. The Dead Cart. A nineteenth-century water-colour based on the fictional description of Daniel Defoe's in *A Journal of the Plague Year*, of dead carts carrying fifteen or sixteen bodies.

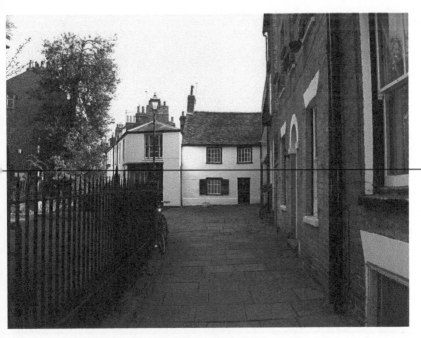

29. Portugal Place, St Clements. Portugal Place overlooks St Clements. It was home to plague victims caught in the second onset of the plague in 1666.

30. Cambridge Bills of Mortality, 31 July to 7 August 1666. This bill was issued during the worse period of infection in 1666.

Cambridge 7.   From July the 31 to *Aug.* the 7th.   1666.

All the Colledges (God be praised) are and have continued without any Infection of the Plague.

	Bur.	Pl.		Bur.	Pl.
St Andrews Cambridge,	10	09	St Giles	00	00
St Andrews Barnwell,	03	03	St Maries Great,	07	05
All-Saints	14	14	St Maries Lesse,	01	01
St Bennetts	06	05	St Michael	01	01
St Botolph	01	01	St Peters	03	02
St Clements	04	04	St Sepulchres	04	04
St Edwards	00	00	Trinity	06	04

The total of Burials in the 14 Parishes this week is —— 60
　Whereof of the Plague ——————— 53
　And at the Pesthouse ———————— 08
　　Increased in the Burials this week ——— 15
　　Whereof of the Plague ————— 11

Fran. Wilford *Vice-chancellour.*   Rowland Simpson *Major.*

31. Cambridge Bills of Mortality, The Final Toll. The bill records the numbers of those who died in the plague of 1665–6, and of those who caught the plague and survived.

There Died in Cambridge of the Plague and of other Diseases from July 1st 1665 to March 19th 1666 ————— 366
　Whereof of the Plague ——————————— 171

A GENERAL BILL
Of all those that have died in Cambridge of the Plague, or of other Diseases, from June the 5th to January the 1. 1666

All the Colledges (God be praised) are and have continued without any Infection of the Plague.

	Bur.	Pla.	Infected Recovered		Bur.	Pla.	Infected Recovered
St Andrews Cambridge,	161	139	160	St Giles	017	013	010
St Andrews Barnwell,	063	031	083	St Maries Great,	048	033	020
All-Saints	097	090	010	St Maries Lesse,	014	011	008
St Bennetts	062	051	013	St Michael	019	013	008
St Botolph	010	013	009	St Peters	012	005	003
St Clements	011	013	006	St Sepulchres	034	017	012
St Edwards	016	006	003	Trinity	153	138	069

The total of Burials in the fourteen Parishes ——————— 758
　Whereof of the Plague ——————————— 594
　　And at the Pesthouse —————————— 155
　In all of the Plague ——————————— 749
　Persons infected that are recovered ——————— 384

The total of Burials in both Visitations ——————— 1124
　Whereof of the Plague —————————— 0910

Francis Wilford *Vice-chancellour.*   John Herring *Major.*

CHAPTER 8

A HARVEST OF DEATH

THE WEATHER IN East Anglia at the beginning of July 1666 was wet, and hailstones threatened the crops ripening in the fields.[1] At least the rain sluiced the streets of Cambridge and kept people indoors, so, they hoped, it would stop the spread of the infection. The weather then turned hot and humid; people complained of head-aches and difficulty in breathing. Towering thunderheads massed over the town, and on 7 July there was a gigantic thunderstorm. Lightning, great rolls of thunder, hail and a strong wind swept the town as the clouds released their massive energy.[2] Children screamed at the noise, people lay on their beds with their fingers in their ears as the lightning crackled and thunder exploded above them. Some counted the interval between the lightning and the crack of the thunder. It was very short. Some prayed that their houses would not be struck by lightning and burnt to the ground, and others that it was not the end of the world. Those who had mirrors covered them up in case they should attract the lightning, others hid in cupboards, under stairs and in cellars. When the storm was over, those who could leave their houses found the streets cleansed by the rain but trees and plants bowed down by the wind.

As well as the houses closed by the plague in June 1666, five more were shut up in the first week of July: those of the Joyces in St Bene't's parish who lived close to Corpus Christi College, the Smiths in Holy Trinity, Widow Tebald, John Fisher, and the Brierleys of All Saints.[3] Richard Joyce came from a family that had lived in St Bene't's from at least 1629 but by quick thinking had avoided paying any rates or taxes.[4] The family survived the plagues of the 1630s and '40s, and in 1652 Richard married Joan Papworth. They had six children, twins Susan and Richard, Mary baptised in 1653, followed by Abigail, who only lived three days, then Thomas, and the youngest, Elizabeth, baptised in 1663.[5] Richard picked up work where he could, but what he preferred to hard labour was drinking in the taverns with his mates, and gambling. He gambled on anything – cockfights, bull baiting, horse and foot races, and in the damp first days of July on which raindrop would reach the bottom of the tavern window first. He was also known by his neighbours to be quick with his fists. He lashed out if someone looked at him or spilt his drink in a tavern, jostled him in the street, or refused to pay up when he had won a bet. In 1660 he was arrested by the university proctors for affray in Barnwell, after he had been to a card game in the Brazen George, and he was not unfamiliar with the inside of the Tolbooth in Petty Cury, or the vice-chancellor's prison.[6] When his daughter Susan fell ill, with what his wife described as a summer cold, Richard made a bargain with God that if Susan merely had a cold and not the plague, he would give up gambling. He was not required to keep his side of the bargain. Susan and her sister Mary died on 3 July, and his son Thomas on the 5th.[7]

Forty-four people died of the plague in the first week of July 1666 and a further 13 were admitted to the pest house. This was bad, but the next week was worse as 77 people in Cambridge died of the plague between 11 and 19 July.[8] Although trade was at a standstill, people had to go about their business, walking past rows of houses with closed doors and the red cross painted across them. Some uttered a prayer for the souls of those inside and for their own preservation as they passed, others crossed their fingers behind their back, or put up two fingers towards the infected houses to ward off evil and the Devil. Mothers dragged their children past the closed doors and refused to answer questions about the red crosses. Friends and relatives of the stricken stood outside in the street and shouted to attract the attention of anyone left alive inside. Once a day the bellman announced the arrival of the dead cart, and the shout of 'Here!' could be heard; the watchmen unlocked the padlock and chain securing the door and the corpse would be passed through. Once a day water and food were brought and the window shutters removed so that the occupants could grab the victuals; if they had any cash left the coins would be dropped into a bowl of vinegar held out by the watch, and whispered requests made for medicine and other necessities.

A walk down Jesus Lane or in Holy Trinity parish at the north end of the Market Place was especially harrowing for passers-by. Six houses in a block were closed up in Holy Trinity, as the infection spread along the row, from Francis Palmer's house where he died on 11 July, to his near neighbour and nephew Samuel Palmer who was buried the next day, and on to Ann Turner's cottage next door, where she died on 14 July. On the other side of Francis Palmer's house Robert Leete, a smith died on the 15th, and Mary Walls on 19 July.[9]

Jesus College stood on the north side of Jesus Lane, and its enclosure took up most of the space on that side. On the south side of the lane were terraces of cottages and tenements. Number 7 Jesus Lane was a divided tenement leased from Jesus College by Thomas Page and sublet to many tenants, all receiving poor relief and exempted from the Hearth Tax.[10] The first death in the tenement was that of Mary, the daughter of Benjamin Dodd an unemployed locksmith, on 6 July. The infection then spread quickly through the tenement. Edward, the son of Daniel and Hannah Claxton, and Susan Turner a deserted wife who had four daughters, and the daughter of Elizabeth Dancer, another deserted wife who lived in a cottage in the tenement's yard, were all buried on 8 July. Two more of the Turner girls died the next day, and Ann Hix, a widow who lived in one room in the tenement, on 10 July. Elizabeth, Benjamin Dodd's wife was buried on 13 July, another of Mrs Dancer's daughters on the 17th, Susan Turner on the 22nd, and Mrs Claxton and her daughter on 30 July. In all, fourteen people died in the tenement and its neighbouring cottage, and two occupants of another shared cottage, Widow Isobel Bletherne and Thomas Gibbs died of the plague on 11 and 20 July, respectively.[11]

Robert Palmer and the Walls family who perished in Holy Trinity parish were also on poor relief and could not pay the Hearth Tax.[12] This led people in Cambridge to look at the overcrowded tenements and shabby cottages of the poor, and shake their heads and mutter that it was the poor who had brought this catastrophe upon the town; but the more rational pointed out that the tenement was close to the common dunghill at the top of Jesus Lane and everyone knew that the plague was caused by bad smells and polluted air, such as came from the dunghill. Those who favoured the poor as the culprits argued that the dwellings of the poor stank; the poor were seen as bringing the infection upon themselves by the conditions in which they lived and by their behaviour and morals. Obviously, they squandered their money in gambling, drunkenness and debauchery – Benjamin Dodd could have got a job if he wanted, and there was no reason why the Walls should have so many children. As the editor of *The Newes* wrote, '. . . the plague is in the sluttish parts of the parish where the poor are crowded together, and the multitude infect one another'.[13]

Was the plague in Cambridge a disease of the poor? 'Poor' needs to be defined, as this is a multifaceted term in the seventeenth century. It could refer to those in receipt of parish relief and excused rates and taxes. It could mean beggars and vagabonds with no fixed abode, who lived on what they could get from charities and other sources. Or it could mean those who lived just at or just below subsistence level, in bad housing, inadequately clothed, and often hungry. Poverty was part of a family's life cycle. Overseers of the Poor Law accounts show that people went in and out of poverty. Young married couples with children too young to earn a living, for example, received relief until the children could go out to work to bolster the family income. Deserted wives such as Susan Turner and Elizabeth Dancer of Jesus Lane, pressed sailors injured in the Dutch War, the soldier maimed in the Civil War, the elderly too frail and sick to work, and widows of all ages appear in Poor Law accounts, but were not all long-term poor.

There is no easy way of estimating the numbers of poor who died in the Cambridge plague outbreaks of 1665 and 1666, and where the occupations of victims have been traced these were usually craftsmen, innkeepers, merchants and at least two gentlemen. They were pillars of the community who served as churchwardens, surveyors of the highways, and overseers of the poor.

Some who died of the plague had not been on poor relief before the plague, but left families who had to apply for relief. The fortunes of one family show poor relief in action. Robert Abelson of Great St Mary's parish died of the plague on 26 July 1666. His orphaned children were taken into care by the parish and lodged out in Coton, Cherry Hinton, and with 'One Cawket' in Little St Mary's parish. The parish provided clothes, shoes and hose for them, and when Robert Abelson junior reached the age of 12 in 1670 he was apprenticed to John Clement a vintner, with the parish paying £8 apprentice duty. Two years later when his sister Susan was apprenticed to Samuel Long, the parish purchased new clothes and shoes for her and paid £6 for her apprenticeship.[14]

Poor relief was given on a sliding scale, pegged to the price of bread and increased by the number of children and dependants the applicant possessed. Even in the seventeenth century this was seen as a system open to abuse, as it was thought to encourage the poor to breed more children in order to increase their benefits. The rate of relief per week varied from 6d to 4s. depending on circumstances. William Clifton and Steven Perry who both died of the plague in August 1666 received poor relief. They lived in houses rented from a property magnate, Troilus Atkinson and the notary Richard Pettit, and part of the relief would have gone straight to their landlords to pay the rent. William Clifton had five children to keep.[15] Illness or injury may have kept him from working, or he may have received injuries fighting the Dutch after being taken by the press in Cambridge. Another large family on poor relief were the Lumpkins of St Bene't's. They had six children and since October 1665 had received 5s. a week to help feed them. Five of these children died of the plague between 9 and 22 August.[16]

The plague had not finished with the occupants of Jesus Lane. Jeremy Reader died on 2 August, and by the 16th his whole family was dead, his sons George, Samuel, Joseph and Daniel and his wife Judith all gone. Reader had moved into Jesus Lane with his family in 1664. His near neighbours included William Watson a shoemaker, and Dr William Floyd who lived at 4 Jesus Lane in the house known as Little Trinity, which stands at the corner of Jesus Lane and Park Street. Today, Little Trinity is a Georgian house built in about 1725, but at the back the seventeenth-century range of timber-framed buildings faced with brick can still be seen, just as they appear on David Loggan's 1688 *Map of Cambridge*.[17]

At the other end of the scale to those on poor relief were those who died of plague but had sufficient property to make a will, or at least a memorandum of their last wishes.[18] The three adult children of Benjamin Lord, a cook, who lived in Great St Mary's parish, all died of the plague; John on 18 July, Obadiah on 19 July and their sister Dorothy on 21 July 1666. Obadiah and Dorothy had sufficient time to make nuncupative wills on their deathbeds. No scribe or lawyer would enter a plague house, so either the instructions were shouted through the window to someone below, or another unfortunate occupant of the house wrote them down.[19]

Obadiah Lord's will is in the form of a memorandum which states that on or about the 19th day of July in the Year of our Lord sixteen sixty-six, Obadiah the eldest son of the late Benjamin Lord cook of Cambridge, being sick in body but of perfect memory made and ordained his last will and testament nuncupative, viz. he gave and bequeathed unto his loving uncle Edward Potto all that he had and all belonging to him, he asked his uncle to pay his debts, and named him sole executor.

Dorothy's will was in a similar form, that of a memorandum. She left her loving father John Blofield a baker (by which she meant her stepfather, as her mother had remarried) all that he had of hers in his hands, and her uncle Edward Potto all that he had of hers in his hands, and also named him as her sole executor. The memorandum did not come to light and go to probate until 17 November 1666. Dorothy's memorandum was witnessed by the wife of William Richardson and Margery Wisdome, so they must have been shut up in the infected house with the Lords. William Richardson had died on 11 July, so it is probable that the Lords were lodging in his house. The Richardsons were related to the Pepys family through William's mother, and were moderately well off, paying 4d a month to the poor rate, and donating 3s. 1d to a special rate for 'the visited shut up in the pest house' levied by the churchwardens of Great St Mary's parish. John Blofield and his wife were both dead before Dorothy's will was proved.[20]

As a cook Benjamin Lord would have left a healthy estate to his children, especially if he was a college cook, as a number of inventories belonging to college cooks indicate that they had possessions worth between £40 and £50.[21] The Lords' stepfather was also a man of property, renting both Chesterton Windmill and the Kings Mills on the Cam by the Little Bridge, opposite to Queens' College. Uncle Edward Potto, their mother's brother, lived in a large house in St Andrew's parish. [22]

Another nuncupative will is that of Daniel Wildman, a mason who lived in Holy Trinity parish. He died of the plague on 21 July 1666; his memorandum was made on 13 July, the day he fell ill, and went to probate on 18 August, after his house came out of quarantine. In his memorandum he left his son Daniel 22s. and his daughters Mary Harper and Ellen Wildman 20s. each. His bonds and bills worth £27, a 5s. golden piece and his pewter dishes were to be divided between his three children. The memorandum was attested as a true account by Adam Sowersby, a church councillor, and John Haughton.[23] This time it was shouted through the window.

Daniel's daughter Mary had married John Harper on 21 September 1665, and they went on to survive the plague and have five children. Her brother Daniel married Mary Towler on 1 October 1665, and their son, another Daniel, was baptised on 12 September 1666. Ellen, the unmarried daughter stayed shut in with their father in his last days, and it is probable that the Ellen Wildman buried on 13 July was her mother.[24]

Masons were a peripatetic group of workmen, moving from job to job. Daniel may have come to Cambridge to work on the new chapel at Peterhouse, completed in about 1665, or on the Wren Chapel or

Hitcham's Cloister at Pembroke College, also completed in 1665.[25] Cambridge was a good place for masons as there was always work going on in the colleges, and this may have prompted Daniel to stay on in the town, especially as his son and daughter had married Cambridge people and he could expect to enjoy his grandchildren in the future. Masons were instantly recognisable in the streets of Cambridge by the stone dust on their clothes, hands and faces, and the paper caps they wore to keep the dust out of their hair. Masons could be layers or setters who built the stone walls, or bankers who worked at their benches to shape the stones. The work at Peterhouse and Pembroke involved facing brick or clunch walls with stone (clunch was a soft chalk building material common to Cambridgeshire.) If Wildman worked at Peterhouse he would have been under the direction of George Thompson, a master mason.[26] Wildman's will suggests that he was a relatively wealthy man, who had saved for the future by investing his money in loans guaranteed by bonds.

Another family who died in the heat of late July and early August of 1666 were the Mauldens of St Andrew's. They were ruled over by the matriarch Alice Maulden, whose husband had long since given up the unequal struggle of life, died and left her moderately well off. She had invested her legacy in buying the lease of three cottages in St Andrew's, and a tenement abutting the highway to Linton and adjoining Ball's Folly Close, which she rented to Samuel Rix, a gentleman.[27] Alice lived in one of the St Andrew's cottages with her son Matthew and grandson Thomas and his family.

Alice's strident tones were familiar in the streets around St Andrew's church, and she was known as someone not to be crossed, as the inspector of beer found out when he arrested her at Stourbridge Fair for selling beer in illegal unmeasured jugs.[28] After a shower of invective and beer, he hauled her off to the fair court, where she was fined 2d. Ma Maulden as she was widely known had seven grandchildren, all grown up by 1666, but living close by and in and out of the family home every day. Ma Maulden ruled her daughter-in-law Matthew's wife with a rod of iron, and when Matthew fell ill she told her daughter-in-law to keep quiet about it. However, someone who had fallen foul of Ma Maulden's tongue in the past told the searchers that there might be plague in her house. When the searchers arrived with their boards, chains, hasps and padlocks Ma Maulden erupted from the house, screaming at them and pummelling them. But she was an old woman, and the searchers and watchmen looked on with amusement, before bundling her back into her house and slamming the door. She was to spend eight weeks inside, as first her son Matthew died on 19 July, then two of her grandchildren on the 20th and 21st, and a day before the quarantine was up her daughter-in-law on 15 August. Ma Maulden survived and emerged in late September.[29]

St Clement's, the epicentre of the plague in 1665, remained clear in the summer of 1666 until Grace, the wife of Samuel North of Portugal Place, died of plague on 15 July. Another inhabitant of Portugal Place, Thomas Coward, died suspected of the plague on 31 July, and his wife Elizabeth on 5 August; another neighbour, George Taylor was taken to the pest house, where he too died.[30] Portugal Place overlooked the churchyard, so its inhabitants would have been very familiar in 1665 with night-time burials in unmarked graves, bobbing lanterns, the chink of shovels on stones, and the soft plop of un-coffined bodies falling into the grave.

The sixteenth-century maps of Cambridge show Portugal Place with houses only on the opposite side of the churchyard, as it is today. The passage led to a pasture where horses and sheep grazed, in close proximity to the King's Ditch. By the seventeenth century another row of houses had been added, backing onto the churchyard, and the pasture had been planted with trees, perhaps an orchard or willow stand. The passage led to St John's College master's dovecote and six fish ponds.[31]

The baking summer days dragged on into August. The colours of Cambridge in that August against a blue or grey sky were the brown of parched grass on the college lawns, Coe Fen and St Thomas's Leys, and the yellow of the corn which stood in the town's West Field, Barnwell Field in the east and the Stourbridge Fair ground. Red poppies added colour in the golden corn, as did the white darnel, that 'pestilent enemy among the corn', growing on borders and pathways of the fields.[32] Despite the weeds it looked like being a good harvest.

Wednesday 1 August was declared a public fast day.[33] A fast in the seventeenth century meant a meatless day. Robert May a seventeenth-century chef to the gentry served sixteen courses on a fast day, starting with oysters, if they were in season, and including buttered eggs on toast, boiled spinach, fish and barley pottage.[34] The inhabitants of Cambridge probably made do with buttered eggs on toast or barley pottage. The ministers might have gone to church to pray on a fast day, but as public assemblies were banned most preferred to spend the day quietly at home or work.

Wednesday was also market day, but few ventured into town from outside to sell their produce. Water, eggs and milk were delivered to the households of wealthier residents who had stayed on in town, but most women did their shopping as speedily as they could, buying bread for their families, passing closed houses with bated breath, and greeting neighbours briefly, fearing to stop for a chat in case they should be infected.

Nine plague victims were buried on 1 August 1666: one each from St Clement's, St Botolph's, All Saints and Holy Sepulchre, two in Great St Mary and three in Holy Trinity.[35] Fifteen deaths followed on 2 August. The plague had taken hold in Great St Mary's parish. On 2 August the whole Lupton family were buried in one grave, Robert Lupton, his wife and four children; and at the same time Abraham Browne's daughters Susanna and Elizabeth were also buried in Great St Mary's churchyard. The Brownes were receiving poor relief and lived in a house owned by the bookseller Edmund Hearne, whose shop and house were on the west side of Great St Mary's church.[36]

Nineteen plague victims were buried between 3 and 5 August, but despite this death toll, life went on. Between 8 July and 26 September 1666, twenty-seven babies conceived during the winter months of 1665 were baptised. Some of these, like Henry, son of John and Elizabeth Leete, who was baptised in Holy Trinity church on 10 September 1666, lost his father to plague on the 23rd of that month and spent the first weeks of his life incarcerated in the infected house with his mother.[37]

Most of the baptisms that took place between July and September 1666 were in St Edward's parish church, which despite its central position and the proximity of plague-stricken Great St Mary remained clear of plague. Six marriages also took place in St Edward's church in the summer of 1666, and two of these were of couples from stricken parishes: Richard Lee and Mary Whitchurch of All Saints parish were married in St Edward's on 14 August and Thomas Morris and Elinor Wildman, of Holy Trinity, married on 9 September.[38]

Baptism meant taking the newborn child to the parish church, and exposing the child to the hazards of the street. Evidence from St Bene't's parish register shows that this took place two to three days after the birth. The mother stayed at home, and the baby was carried to church either by the godparents or by a specially designated elderly woman known as the godsip, who had no blood relationship to the family. This was to prevent any future match between people within the forbidden degrees of consanguinity, as according to folklore whoever carried the child to church to be baptised was believed to be related to that child. Then as now, the service at the font was a sacrament: it welcomed the baby into the Church, demonstrated the faith of the parents, and set out the obligations of the godparents; and it was often the godparents who chose the name. The baby's name and the father's name were then entered in the parish register.

The baby usually cried as the sign of the Cross was made with holy water on its forehead. This was seen as a good sign, as it meant the Devil had been ejected, and was applauded by those present. After the service the baby was returned to the mother and there would be some modest feasting, and 'wetting the baby's head' with ale or wine. In the summer of 1666 baptism was a hurried affair, with a small group of people gathered round the font, and then quickly home to prevent the infected plague air getting to the baby.

The religious aspect of childbearing did not stop there. The Book of Common Prayer of 1603 decreed that a month after childbirth the mother should be churched, or purified in the parish church. This might be a ceremony with family and friends present, or consist of a solitary woman sitting by herself.[39] Whether this took place or not might depend on the enthusiasm of the parson for ritual and liturgy, and the willingness of the woman to conform. In the plague months of 1666 it would have been abandoned.

Even in plague time, marriages could be a joyous affair. At the height of the plague in London, on 28 August 1666, Samuel Pepys attended Mr Longracke's wedding, and the reception afterwards in the Philpott Lane cook shop, where there was 'Good dinner and good music. Dancing.'[40]

In Cambridge many marriages took place in the early morning so that the couple did not lose a day's work, but the reception took place in the evening and, depending on the finances of the couple, might include a full meal with wine, or cakes and ale. Dancing would follow, and the couple would retire to bed with much ribaldry, rude songs and gestures from their friends. Marriages in plague-ridden Cambridge were more sombre affairs – a hasty ceremony and no celebrations – although promises were made that when the plague had abated there would be great feasting.

The plague could not stop people falling in love. Thirty-three marriages took place in the winter of 1666–67, of couples who had fallen in love during the plague and had had to wait until it was declared 'all clear'. One bride was Lizzie Twells of Holy Sepulchre, who met Thomas Ashby a barge-master from King's Lynn when she was on the Quayside in April 1666. He took her for a drink in the nearby Ship Inn, and they fell in love. His barge, with its brown sail patched in red, brought coal down the river from King's Lynn and loaded up with malt from the malt house in St Clement's, or wheat from the West Field, for the return journey. The round trip took up to a month so Lizzie knew roughly when to expect him and would be waiting at the Quayside. In June 1666, King's Lynn corporation forbade all communication with the town of Cambridge, and so the couple were left to wait, Thomas not knowing if Lizzie had been infected and died of the plague, and Lizzie wondering if Thomas would remain faithful to her.

Another couple who fell in love in the spring of 1666, when it seemed as if the worst for Cambridge was over, were Thomas Redhead aged 20 of St Andrew the Great parish, and Mary Priest of Little St Mary's, who had met when Thomas, apprenticed to William Crane a scrivener, had delivered some property deeds to her father.[41]

Thomas Redhead lived in a modest house with his father Robert, his stepmother, two baby stepsisters, his grandmother and his aunt. It was an overcrowded but exuberant household, and nearby were his uncle Henry and his cousin Elizabeth, the two families visiting each other and sharing meals. Thomas might be shabby and ink-stained but he had ambition to emulate his master, and make a fortune investing in the bonds and mortgages that he had written.

Selection meant that the red hair of the original Redheads had calmed down, but they still retained the pale skin of the redhead, and Thomas had a propensity to burn, so that in the hot summer sun his face was red and peeling. Mary would soothe it with a salve of camomile, and as her cool fingers stroked his face Thomas thought he was the luckiest man alive. Their courtship was not to run smoothly. On Midsummer Day, when Thomas had intended to take Mary to the fair, his grandmother fell ill with a fever. She died of the plague on 24 June, and his aunt on 12 July. Thomas was shut up in the plague house, and relied on his neighbour Cuthbert Patteson to take word to Mary, and tell her he still loved her.[42]

There were fifty-three plague burials in total in the first week of August, and eight people admitted to the pest house.[43] Not unexpectedly, the royal proclamation banning Stourbridge Fair arrived in the town on 6 August.[44]

Some of those who had escaped the plague in 1665 now began to succumb to infection. The family of Peter Lightfoot the fishmonger, who lived in St John's Lane in St Clement's parish, had counted themselves lucky to have survived in 1665, but when their daughter Sara died suspected of the plague on 6 August, they knew the worst had happened. Sara's sister Joyce died on 23 August, three-year-old Ann on 11 September, their grandmother, seven-year-old Richard and four-year-old Elizabeth were all buried on 21 September, and just when it looked as if there would be no more deaths, and they could come out of quarantine, Peter's apprentice John Sell died of the plague on 23 October 1666. The family spent four months incarcerated in their house, shut up with the dead and dying. Peter, his wife Joyce, and his son Peter were the only survivors, but in March 1667 a baby girl named Joyce for her mother and her dead sister was baptised, and a year later, in June 1668, a son, another Richard, was also baptised.[45]

Peter Lightfoot had to struggle to regain the trade he had lost, and his position in society as a freeman and burgess, bailiff of the Tolbooth, and a common council man. It took until 1688 for him to advance to become an alderman, when the corporation was purged by a Royal Commission. He lived in a substantial house with eight rooms, but his next door neighbour was Felix Woodward, whose daughter Ann had died of the plague in January 1666, so there were infected rats and blocked fleas in the area, travelling between houses via the roof spaces.

A quirk of parish boundaries meant that Cambridge Castle lay in Chesterton parish, and it is possible that the plague victims in Chesterton came from the cottages by the castle. Those who succumbed included Philip, son of Robert and Dorothy Johnson, and the Doughty family. Joseph the father died of plague on 10 August, followed by his wife Margaret and his son Joseph on 23 August, and another son Thomas on 29 August.[46]

By mid-August in the fields surrounding Cambridge the corn was ripe and ready, when it turned wet.[47] The farmers desperately needed to get their crops in before it rotted in the fields, but with so many houses shut up, labour was scarce. A group of men who leased land on Barnwell Field – John Adams, John Danks a college cook, and four shoemakers, Henry Atkinson, John Jenkinson, Joseph Gascoigne and Thomas Glover[48] – met in the Brazen George to discuss what could be done, and how much they were prepared to offer to entice labour into the fields. The usual daily rate for a labourer in harvest was 1s. 6d, but this was increased during harvest time. Henry Atkinson suggested doubling it, and they eventually settled on 2s. 6d a day, but word on the streets of Cambridge was that they were offering 7s. a day, and this rumour reached London: 'At Cambridge it [the plague] is so sore that the harvest can hardly be gathered in, though 7s. a day is offered.'[49]

Some of the labour force the Barnwell farmers needed for harvest were agricultural specialists: reapers who cut the wheat, bending over the crop and using a short-handled sickle, or mowers who cut barley and oats with a long-handled scythe, standing upright and working in a line across the field.[50] A large number of unskilled labourers followed the reapers, for wheat had to be tied into sheaves and stacked into stooks to dry, and trains of wagons and horses with loaders were then needed to collect the sheaves from the field and take them into storage.

In the last act of the harvest the women and children were allowed on to the field to collect grain that had been dropped. This was of inestimable value to the household budget, and could keep the family in bread for months. Eventually, the high wages offered meant that the Barnwell fields were harvested, and a few brave women went into the fields to glean. Despite this, the yield for 1665 and 1666 was lower than expected, perhaps because of the wet period in late August, and prices were high,[51] creating an additional burden on the poor and the poor rate.

This episode shows that although Cambridge had all the trappings of a town – a corporation and civic life, high density of population, and many goods and services on offer – it was still tied to the countryside. The lessees of the fields surrounding the town and the burgesses who grazed cattle and sheep on Coe Fen and Midsummer Common, who took grain to be milled at the King's Mills or Chesterton Windmill, were tradesmen and professionals whose daily life was based on an urban economy. But anyone who climbed to the roof of King's College Chapel in August 1666 would have seen the town surrounded by a sea of wheat, with islands of pasture dotted with animals.

Those aldermen who had not fled, or who dared to come back to town, met at a subdued Common Day (Town Council) meeting on 16 August to elect John Herring a draper as mayor for the next year.[52] No sugar cakes or wine followed the meeting, and the new mayor gave no dinner to celebrate his election; instead, the aldermen scuttled away as fast as they could, holding scarves to their faces or sniffing pomanders to keep the deadly air away.

The last week of August saw 35 plague burials and 16 people sent to the pest houses.[53] Twenty-two of the plague burials were in Holy Trinity parish, including those of six members of the Palmer family. They had been on poor relief and lived crammed into one room and an attic, next door to another poor family the Bowmans, who lost four family members, and the Beetons who lived in a court off Shoemakers' Row, which had been created by in-filling yards with two-roomed cottages built of wattle and daub and with thatched roofs; perfect places for the plague to prosper.[54]

Poor or not, family was important in the seventeenth century. Harrowing as it was to tend dying family members, at least they did not die alone but in the arms of their loved ones, and those who survived could mourn together and give and take what cheer they could. When they eventually emerged from quarantine they could rebuild their lives together. In the months of July and August, forty-one Cambridge families were directly affected by the plague.

CHAPTER 9

THE BEGINNING OF THE
END OF THE PESTILENCE

SUNDAY 2 SEPTEMBER was warm and dry, pleasant weather which encouraged Cambridge people to venture out of doors and stroll by the river or on Midsummer Common. In the churches prayers were offered for those stricken with the plague, and for peace with the Dutch who were rumoured to be off the East Anglian coast, and there were signs in London and Colchester that the pestilence might be abating. That evening there were other more pressing concerns in London. A fire started in a baker's shop in Pudding Lane, spread and burned brightly for days, destroying some 13,000 houses and making at least 100,000 people homeless. St Paul's Cathedral was gutted, as well as 84 parish churches, the Guildhall, the Royal Exchange and 52 livery company halls. The square mile of the City of London was totally destroyed. This became known as the Great Fire of London; luckily only a few citizens perished.[1]

The news reached Cambridge by 9 September and was transmitted to Samuel Newton, still in exile in Waterbeach. He had not written in his diary since 3 January 1666, but now he felt compelled to get out his diary again, blow off the dust and pen the following account.

On Sunday morning between one and 2 of the clock in the morning in the City of London a fire began in Pudding Lane at a french bakers [sic] house to be fired [sic] (and it being a great north west wind) continued most fiercely burning from that time until Thursday in the afternoon being the 6th day of September. It burned down ... parishes with churches and consumed all along from where it began to the Tower, and also towards Westminster as far as Temple Bar. Not above 2 or 3 persons that were consumed by fire, and for light commodities and which were of most value, most persons got them away into the fields, but at such vast rates for carriage 8 or 10 pounds for the carriage of a load of goods was ordinarily given.[2]

Newton had received some but not all of the details of the fire. He did not know how many parishes and parish churches had been destroyed, but he did know how much people were paying to evacuate their goods, which suggests that this aspect was of some concern to the person or newspaper that had provided him with the information. Newton stayed on in Waterbeach for the time being, since Cambridge was still infected; death in one family, the Frohocks, brought the plague close to him as they were his cousins. Samuel and John Frohock were butchers and graziers.[3] Samuel sold meat from two stalls in the Shambles and grazed cattle out on the Fens at Aldreth near Haddenham, and although he had a house in Shoemakers' Row, he also had one at Aldreth; during the plague he departed to live there. John stayed on in Cambridge. He had a lease on a mansion house called Michaelhouse Grange, and grazing on what is now Parker's Piece, land in Barnwell Field, the West Field, and Trumpington Field.[4] He lived in Little St Mary's parish, and it was there that his daughter Mercy died of the plague on 1 September 1666.[5]

John Frohock had four other children, all under ten years old. When Mercy fell sick, he did what he thought was best for them: bundled them into a cart, covered them with sacks and drove them to Fulbourn six miles south-west of Cambridge, where his cousin Francis lived.[6] The journey took a day as he made detours to avoid roadblocks set by villages, where visitors from infected Cambridge were not welcome. When he was close to Fulbourn he hid the cart and his children on Fulbourn Fen and went on foot into the village, carefully avoiding the farm owned by Queens' College, where refugee college fellows might be living, and found his cousin. It took an hour of pleading and the promise of £20 before Francis would agree to take the children, but eventually he did and under cover of darkness John wrapped each child in a sack and carried them one by one to his cousin's house. Wearily, he returned to his cart, and to Cambridge, but when, in the pale light of dawn, he saw the red cross on his house door and watchmen waiting for him outside, he drove on. Reasoning that it was better for one parent to survive to care for the children, he moved in with his brother Samuel at Aldreth. He was reunited with his wife and children on 10 October 1666.

Thomas Redhead, the scrivener's apprentice peered disconsolately out of the windows of his father's house. The warmth of the early September sun was unbearable and he yearned to get away from the smell of death, fouled bedding, dirty pots and pans; he longed to strip off his clothes and plunge into the cool and cleansing river. The hearths in the house stood empty, and Thomas and his father existed on bread and water. Thomas hoped that Mary Priest was well and would remember him, but lethargy was setting in and he could do little more than sit with his head in his hands. Similarly, Lizzie Twells received no news from King's Lynn about her lover, and up in King's Lynn, clear of the plague, Thomas Ashby was equally worried.

Twenty-five houses were closed up in the first week of September. Eight were in the small parish of St Michael's, where houses were on the High Street or in closes behind it. Timothy Caverley lived in one of the small houses that stood on the High Street, and until 1664 his 30-year-old son Thomas had lived next door. But in 1665 he had married and moved to one of the closes behind the High Street.[7] The Caverleys were locksmiths. This was a trade which required the knowledge of two skills: ironwork and smithing to produce lock plates and keys, and a delicate touch to manipulate the mechanism of the lock.

Cambridge was a town of locks. There were fifteen different locks on doors in King's College Chapel, ranging from locked bars which secured external doors, to iron boxes with locks inside the chapel.[8] There were locks on college gates, locks on the university chest, and three locks on each parish chest, which required the minister and two churchwardens to open it. The parish chest contained the parish register and other civic documents, and behind the locked door of the vestry was the church plate, which could be very extensive. St Mary the Great's church plate included two great silver flagons given to the church by John Crane a town benefactor, and two silver bowls with covers. The poorer parish of Holy Trinity's vestry contained a silver and gilt cup dated 1569, another dated 1622, and two pewter flagons. In 1666 the official keyholders of Holy Trinity church were John Leyton, Francis Challis and John Turkington, each of whom held two keys, one to unlock the vestry and one to unlock the parish chest.[9]

When he was a student at Trinity College, Isaac Newton purchased a lock for his desk for 1s. 4d and another for his study costing 1s. 8d.[10] Servants kept their personal possessions in locked boxes and chests, shopkeepers kept their takings in locked boxes, ladies locked away their jewellery, and important family documents were kept in locked document boxes. Samuel Newton and his legal colleagues kept their offices locked, their front doors locked with an iron key, and barred and locked from the inside at night. College bursars had ranks of locked boxes in the college muniments rooms and in the bursary.[11]

Locksmiths should have made a good living, but the work was spasmodic. New builds needed locks, joiners purchased locks to put on the boxes, chests and trunks they made, but much of the work was in repairing old locks, replacing lost keys, and opening doors when keys were lost. There was little new building in Cambridge during the 1660s, and only one of the fifteen locks in King's College Chapel is seventeenth-century.[12] Most of the college locks had been fitted centuries earlier. The Caverleys lived on the edge of poverty, and to boost their income sold beer at the Midsummer and Stourbridge Fairs. Both Timothy and Thomas had been arrested for selling false measures of beer at Stourbridge Fair in 1664.[13] When Thomas married he moved out of the family home and into another cottage in St Michael's parish. As a plague preventive the two families decided to keep apart and so it was Thomas's new neighbour Henry Chandler who came to tell Timothy that Thomas's cottage and workshop had been closed for three days and nobody had seen Thomas or his wife, and it was Thomas's sister Sarah who went to the house, knocked on the door and peered through the windows. When she tried to push the door open she found something wedged behind it. Eventually she found an un-shuttered window and squeezed through it. She found her brother lying on the floor behind the front door, full of plague tokens. Telltale black blains were on his face and arms, buboes under his armpits; his lips were dry and cracked, and he gave an occasional death rattle. The house smelt of decay, faeces and vomit. Sarah moistened his lips and tried to clean him up, but he died a few hours later on 7 September 1666.[14] His was the last death from plague in St Michael's parish.

Other parishes were not so fortunate. In the second week of September there were eighteen plague deaths in Holy Trinity, four each in St Giles and St Mary the Great, and one each in St Bene't and St Clement; a further eleven people were sent to the pest house.[15] One of those who died that week in Holy Trinity was Joseph Gascoigne a cordwainer, who lived in Shoemakers' Row. The word cordwainer comes from the Cordova leather used for high-quality shoes and boots, so Gascoigne was at the high-end luxury market. Some idea of the cost of shoes in seventeenth-century Cambridge comes from Isaac Newton, who paid 4s. for each pair he purchased in Cambridge, plus 2s. for shoelaces, and 10d to have his shoes mended.[16]

Gascoigne was a burgess with a booth at Stourbridge Fair, and he had invested some of his capital in property with leases on land in Fair Yard Lane, on Barnwell Field, a tenement in Great St Mary's parish, a house in Slaughter House Lane and another in Shoemakers' Row, as well as property at Longstow in the Fens. He was well known in Holy Trinity parish, serving as churchwarden in 1641, 1649 and 1658, and as parish councillor in 1660, 1662, 1663 and 1666.[17]

He made his will on 24 July 1666, perhaps as insurance against the future as the plague was already rife in Cambridge. He left his loving wife Joan the house where they lived in Shoemakers' Row, with its yard and gardens, for her life-time and then to pass to his son Joseph. Joseph junior was to pay his sister Elizabeth £40 on the day of her marriage or within twelve months thereof and she was to have the booth at Stourbridge Fair called Soper's House and all the timber and tilts that went with it, and two timber booths at Barnwell for ever, but his wife Joan was to have the profits from these for life. Elizabeth was also bequeathed the lease of a property in Slaughter House Lane, and again Joan was to receive the profits from this for her life-time. All the remainder was to go to his wife, who was to pay his debts, and she was to be an executor with his son and daughter.[18] The will suggests that Gascoigne's wife and daughter were left better off than his son, but it is likely that the major share of the inheritance and the cordwaining business had been given to his son before the will was made. Joseph Gascoigne senior died of the plague on 9 September and his loving wife Joan on 21 September. No inventory exists for his house and shop, but the latter would have included leather worth anything between £30 and £100, as well as his shoe-making implements, shoe lasts, and any shoes already made.

The full count of plague deaths from 4 to 11 September was 32, with five people admitted to the pest house, while from 11 to 18 September a further 19 people died of the plague and six more went to the pest house. On 23 September the corporation renewed its order forbidding public assemblies and cancelled the annual mayoral dinner again.[19]

Among those who died in this period were Alderman Mr Richard Allan, a vintner of Great St Mary's, and Matthew, Piers and Charles, the sons of Edward Bird, aged 16, 10 and 7 who were also buried. The Birds were a living example to many of their neighbours of how poor relief encouraged the poor to breed, as Edward and Dorcas Bird had ten children, eight of whom survived infancy.[20] Thomasine, the wife of James Blackley who rented the Water Fair ground died on 29 August. James, shut up in their house, made his will on 7 September daily expecting to die. He asked to be buried beside Thomasine. He gave John and Robert Rybread the lease of the house where he lived; his son James Blackley was to have £40 a year from the profits of the Hanging Bird Bolt Inn in St Andrew's Street and his father's wearing apparel. Thomasine's wearing apparel was to go to their daughter Elizabeth Bennet, with 20s. of money, and the rest of his goods were for his son John, who was to pay his daughter Mary 20s. and discharge his father's debts as his executor. As an afterthought he added that his son

Matthew was to receive 5s. within five months of his father's death.[21] Matthew Blackley was the black sheep of the family. James Blackley was a Quaker and Parliamentarian who had spent time in the Castle Gaol for his beliefs.[22] Matthew, a baker by trade, was rumoured to be a recusant, which meant he had converted to Catholicism, perhaps as an act of rebellion against his father. He appeared in the session court on a charge of breach of the peace, and was described as a privileged person of the university, and bound over. Much later in the seventeenth century his name reached James II as that of a person who could take the cause of Catholicism into the countryside, and in 1688 James sacked Cambridge Corporation and made Matthew Blackley its mayor. Those who lost office included Samuel Newton.[23]

As September drew to a close the air grew moist, and sowing the seed for the following year's crop was threatened. On 30 September there was a great storm, with furious winds blowing all night. October came in with floods. The Cam overflowed its banks, water lay in sheets on the Fens, and a cold rain fell.[24] There were thirty-six plague burials in Cambridge in the last weeks of September and the beginning of October, five people were admitted to the pest houses, and during September St Peter's parish carried to the pest houses another fifteen people, who died there.[25]

Conditions in the pest houses on Coldham Common and Jesus Green were such that few ventured near them, and to be taken there was almost certain death. Masked attendants delivered food and drink to the stricken, who usually died alone, far from family and friends and calling out for help, and were then shovelled into pits. The apothecaries who remained in town sent in distilled waters and salves to help the infected.

Artemus Hinde who lived in St Giles watched the pathetic bundles from St Peter's parish being thrown into carts to be taken to the pest house. William Frisby who lived in Great St Mary's parish was surrounded by the plague, and Peter Dent saw his neighbours' houses shut up and the red cross painted on the door close to his shop next to the Holy Sepulchre church. Peter Dent was lucky as he could escape to his physic garden and smell sweet herbs, touch cool plants and breathe in pure fresh air. He could busy himself in his still room, teach his son the properties of plants and minerals, and for a while escape the horrors of the world outside.[26]

In Impington, a village just to the north of Cambridge, plague arrived on 30 September 1666 when John Heward died and was buried 'on the moor' by his wife and a maidservant. His daughter Mary died on 9 October and was buried by the maidservant, and on 30 October Mary Everett died of the 'supposed' plague and was buried in the field next to her grandfather's house by her grand-mother and mother. These pathetic burials in unconsecrated ground by family members add a new horror to the plague: the women of the families being forced to dig the grave and between them carry the corpses to their burying place. Did they whisper some approximation of the burial service over the departed?[27]

Thomas Redhead endured being shut up in the infected house with his father and stepmother for the whole of September; they no longer talked, but eyed each other warily, looking for plague tokens. Thomas took a kitchen knife and cut notches in a beam above the empty hearth: one for each day, and a cross bar to show that five days had elapsed. As the line began to grow he could count 35 and then 38 days since his sister Elizabeth's death. Then at last, on 4 October, came the welcome sound of the boards being levered off the door and whitewash obliterating the red cross. All he wanted to do now was to wash and get clean clothes, and make sure that his Mary had also survived the plague and still loved him. Thomas Redhead and Mary Priest were married in the parish church of St Andrew the Great on 27 February 1667. Their son Thomas was baptised in the same church on 25 October 1668, followed by a daughter Mary on 20 February 1670.[28]

The continual rain in October turned the roads into quagmires, but despite this, the near cessation of the plague in London meant that communication between the capital and Cambridge started again. The coach service resumed, and coaches and carriers' carts brought in longed-for letters, newspapers, and information about life in London society and new fashions. Pepys and Evelyn both mentioned a new fashion for men: the 'Vest' (a sort of waistcoat). Pepys, who first saw it at court on 17 October 1666, remarked that 'the court is full of vests'. Evelyn saw it the day after, at the Court of Star Chamber. He thought that the fashion was of Persian origin. He had his own vest and tunic to wear on 30 October. Pepys got his on 4 November. Tailors in London began making vests to order, and the carriers brought sketches of these for the Cambridge tailors to copy. Isaac Newton decided to follow fashion and have a vest of his own. He paid £2 for two yards of worsted prunella and a buckle to be made into a vest.[29]

On a more sombre note, a fast and collection for those displaced by the Great Fire of London were held on 10 October, and in Cambridge plague victims were still being buried. However, the numbers were going down with only seven buried in the first ten days of October; but now families who so far had escaped were infected. Barbary and John Rogers of Great St Mary who had only been married three years, and still waited hopefully for a child, and John Fitch a baker and his daughter Lydia all died in the first days of October.

On the 13th, Samuel Newton, still out at Waterbeach, saw a strange phenomenon in the sky, and wrote about it in his diary:

Saturday 13th October from 5 to about half an hour after 6 at night the north west part of the heavens (in my thoughts) seemed many times to burn and be all of a red fire, it came after the manner of lightning but the flashes were more red (even of fire) also much larger and of longer continuance, there were also 2 small thunder claps which with a tempest did over turn many houses and the greatest part of a church.[30]

Those who saw this unnatural storm in Cambridge wondered if it heralded the end of the world, but the learned reassured them that it could not be so, as the end of the world would start in the east. This was no comfort to George and Ann Overton, shut up in their house in St Andrew's after the death of their sister Sarah. They covered their eyes and cringed in a corner away from the windows; Surely God or the Devil had come to get them. Ann and Mary Thompson who lived in Holy Trinity parish were already in the final stages of the plague; they grew delirious and Ann found the strength to rise from her bed and run howling round the room, banging on doors and windows while the storm raged outside.[31]

On 26 October Samuel Newton deemed it safe to leave Waterbeach and return to his house by St Edward's church in Cambridge. He had been away four months, and he found the town much changed. Quieter: the students would normally have returned by this time. Subdued: there were no civic processions and no dinners to attend, and there were still red crosses on doors in the streets, while the last week of October saw a further nine plague burials in the town. Samuel Newton may have regretted his return from the countryside, as he recorded on 1 November, 'On Thursday died Peter Thurloe's wife of the sickness'. Peter Thurloe lived close to him in St Edward's parish.[32]

St Edward's parish register does not record any plague deaths in the parish, but the Bills of Mortality do note twelve from June 1665 to March 1666, four in July 1666, and one each in September and November.[33] Either the parish clerk was being economical with the truth by leaving plague deaths out of the register, a practice not unknown in the seventeenth century, or these victims died in the pest house, their names unlisted but their parish of origin recorded.

Barges began to arrive from King's Lynn at the end of October, and Lizzie Twells haunted the Quayside in the hope that the barge with the patched brown sail would reappear. On 31 October, when dead souls rise and Sibell Merrifield died of the plague in Holy Trinity parish, she saw the familiar sail coming down the river. She married Thomas Ashby, the barge-master from King's Lynn, in her home parish of Holy Sepulchre on 28 January 1667.[34] Lizzie left on the barge, cleaned and decorated with green boughs and hollies, to start a new life in another town.

November started with good weather, but on the 11th of that month turned wet and dirty. In Cambridge there was a rumour that London was on fire again, but it turned out to be no more than fires still smouldering in the ruins, or squatters lighting fires to keep themselves warm. There had been a real alarum on 9 November when fire broke out in Whitehall, and the whole city was in uproar thinking this was a French invasion, but it turned out to be a fire in the king's stables.[35]

There were eight plague deaths in Cambridge that November. Hannah Woods from Holy Trinity, Christianne Howell and Elizabeth Clothier in St Andrew's, Francis Hill's son in St Giles, Annis Inman of St Mary the Less, an unnamed person from St Peter's in the pest house, and on 28 November Abraham Masterson and his wife were buried in the churchyard of St Mary the Great.[36] But life was slowly returning to normal. On 20 November Samuel Newton attended the wedding in King's College Chapel of William Wells a vintner to Jane Allen, the widow of Richard Allen another vintner, who had died of the plague. William Wells was Samuel Newton's near neighbour.[37] This marriage shows that people directly affected by the plague were beginning to make choices about how they would spend the rest of their lives.

There were three plague deaths in the first three weeks of December. Two in St Andrew's and one in All Saints parish, and then the Bill of Mortality for the last week of December revealed there were no further deaths from plague.[38] The town was clear.

Although there were still eleven red crosses on doors, the pestilence was over. The town could return to normal. The colleges could open their doors again, the students could return, lectures could begin. Some townsfolk went to church to pray for those who had died, and on Christmas Day 1666 many took communion for the first time in a year. The corporation was back in business, regular meetings resumed, apprentices were given their freedom by the corporation, and the Regent House, the university's governing body, went into session.[39]

Inns and cook shops reopened. There was fresh produce in the market, neighbours stopped to gossip again, children were allowed out into the streets to play and run errands, and the noise of work and social commerce was heard. But there was still a subdued air about the town, as if it was dazed and in shock. Many did not know what to do, or how to wake up to the New Year. So many familiar faces were missing, and there were so many raw earthen graves in the churchyards. The survivors sometimes felt guilty, and those who had lost family and friends to the pestilence continued to mourn. Samuel Pepys summed up the year at the end of his diary for 1666: 'Thus ends this year of public wonder and mischief to this nation – and therefore generally wished by all people to be at an end.'[40] A sentiment with which those living in Cambridge during the years 1665 and 1666 would have heartily agreed.

CHAPTER 10

THE FINAL TOLL

THE FINAL TOLL of plague deaths given in the Cambridge Bills of Mortality was 920 burials in churchyards and pest house plague pits. This number included Barnwell, for which there is no other information.[1] It amounts to 12 per cent of the population of the town. Although nowhere near the 100,000 deaths in London or 2,000 in Colchester, because Cambridge was much smaller it nevertheless meant that almost everyone knew someone who had died of plague, or of an infected family in a closed house. Unusually, the Cambridge final Bill of Mortality gives the number of people who were suspected of having been infected by the plague and of having recovered as 384 souls, which meant that 1,304 people or 16 per cent of the population were directly affected by the plague.

The seventeenth-century statistician Sir William Petty suggested that in London 'let the mortality be what it will, the city repairs its loss of inhabitants within two years'.[2] This optimism was based on an inflated baptismal rate in the months following the plague. While this may have been true for London, smaller towns could suffer years of demographic stagnation after a cataclysmic event such as the plague.[3] The Hearth Tax returns for Cambridge show a drop of 269 entries for the decade between 1664 and 1674, a loss of 14 per cent.[4] This suggests that the population was struggling to regain its pre-plague level, despite incomers from the countryside migrating into the town. In terms of actual population figures, using a multiple of 4.5 on the Hearth Tax returns suggests a population of 8,744 in 1664 and 7,533 in 1674. The lower figure is confirmed by an ecclesiastic census taken by Bishop Compton in 1676 of all communicants, Nonconformists and Catholics. It is assumed that the census refers to all those over the age of 16, and a multiple of 2.5 to account for the total population of Cambridge suggests that the figure is about 7,007.[5]

In Cambridge only All Saints and Holy Trinity parishes showed no loss of population between 1664 and 1674; all the other parishes showed losses, from 27 per cent at St Andrew the Great to 1 per cent in St Mary the Great. The town's population had not recovered from the plague. This is borne out by the parish registers. There was no great rush of marriages after the plague, and no inflation of baptisms, and the numbers of these events did not reach pre-plague levels until the late 1670s.

Behind the figures were people. Of those who died of plague whose ages can be traced 70 per cent were adults and 30 per cent children. There was a different pattern of deaths in other towns such as Colchester or Norwich, where children were the hardest hit.[6] In Cambridge most of the child deaths came in the first onslaught of the plague in 1665. Of the adults, 41 per cent were men, and 49 per cent were women. Many of the women were single, and were probably young women who had moved from the country to the town to find employment in the colleges, and as servants in inns and town houses.

At least twenty-nine whole families were wiped out by the plague. Seventeen husbands were left with children to look after when their wives died of the plague, and ten wives were left with children when their husbands died. Ten married couples died. Family life and households were disrupted by the plague. There were spaces never to be filled at the hearth and in the heart, but some remarried quickly, such as Francis Bird's widow Ann who married William Sell in December 1665 so that they could reopen the Ship Inn together, or Nicholas Rabber, whose wife Margaret died of the plague, who remarried in December 1667.[7]

Some families who had lost children in the plague replaced them in the following years. Elias Woodward baptised a son in 1667, and Lancelot Hooper was blessed with a daughter in 1668; Benjamin Dodd who lived in the Jesus Lane tenement baptised a son in 1667 and a daughter in 1668.

Plague had disrupted everyday life. Communication had been difficult between Cambridge and its nearby villages, and between Cambridge and London. When the plague finally ceased relationships had to be re-established, and people had to find out what had happened to their friends and family. In Cambridge once the plague was deemed over, the searchers and the watchmen who had had to enforce the Plague Orders, nail shut doors, chase and capture those who fled from infected houses, and send the sick to the pest houses faced an uneasy future. Vivid recollections of these individuals and their role during the plague would stay in folk memory for many years, and could make their lives and those of their children very difficult.[8]

The economic toll was high as well. Two watchmen for every infected house, as stated in the Plague Orders, cost 16d a day for each house.[9] In the early days of the plague it might have been possible to fulfil this order, but as the number of infected houses grew, the strain on manpower and finances means this was probably discontinued. From July to September 1665, for example, 34 houses were closed, requiring 68 watchmen to stand outside, at a cost in total of £9 6s. a day, and some houses were in quarantine for at least 40 days at a cost of £372 per house. The Plague Orders also allocated 8d a day for each infected person for victuals, fuel and medicine.[10] As 1,304 people were infected with plague, this meant a total of at least £43 9s. 6d a day. It is true that many victims survived only one or two days after infection, and the costs are spread over two years, but had the order been adhered to the town would have been bankrupt. There is no record of payments made by victims to the watchmen, other than those taken from the parish poor rates, and the special rate levied by Great St Mary's parish.

Trade and industry had been almost at a standstill in Cambridge during the plague, but now they had to re-start, and those craftsmen who had been affected by the plague, such as Christopher Bumstead the brazier or John Bullin the hat-maker, had to find the capital to buy raw materials, and regain their custom. Publicans, cook-shop owners, bakers and confectioners had all suffered financially and had to rebuild their businesses when the plague was over. Some towns, Liverpool for example, compensated tradesmen whose businesses were closed due to suspected infection,[11] but there is no record of this for Cambridge.

Corporation business reopened in November 1666 when Thomas Wendy, the baker William Kelsey's son-in-law, who had been apprenticed to his father James Wendy, butcher, was freed, and on 11 January 1667 Thomas Nicholson apprenticed to John Bird, blacksmith was freed, as were Thomas Glover the apprentice of his father Thomas a cordwainer, and Robert Crabb another cordwainer, who had been apprenticed to Christopher Symonds.[12] They had survived the plague and worked through it. In 1667 the mayoral elections and feasts resumed when public notary Richard Pettit was elected mayor, followed in 1668 by Nathaniel Crabbe for a second term of office, and in 1671 by Samuel Newton.[13]

Samuel Newton had returned from his self-imposed exile in Waterbeach in October 1666 to take up his life again. On 12 February 1667 he enrolled his son John aged eight in the Grammar Free School on the recommendation of Dr Robert Brady, master of Caius College.[14] The assizes returned to the town in March, and Garlic Fair was held for the first time in two years on 15 August, followed by – to the relief of town and university – Stourbridge Fair. In October the custom of visiting the new mayor and partaking of sack and sugar cakes resumed, and Samuel Newton was chosen to become a common councilman in the place of Mr Edward Potto, the uncle of the Lord siblings Obadiah and Dorothy who had died in the plague. To celebrate his election Samuel invited the other twenty-four councilmen, the town clerk and town attorneys back to his house for sack purchased from Owen Mayfield's inn the Mitre, and accompanied by the university musicians whom Newton had hired for the occasion.

Newton's first year following the plague ended on a sombre note, as on 20 December his wife Sarah had 'a most grievous fit of the stone colic, which held her all that day and the next, insomuch as that I feared her death, but God be pleased to deliver her'.[15] His life at this time was not without tragedy as his infant son Samuel, born on 27 September 1668 and baptised in St Edward's church on 4 October, died on 26 March 1669.[16]

Samuel Newton's civic career was to rise meteorically. In August 1668 he became an alderman, and in September 1671 he was elected mayor. In his inaugural speech he signified 'How in my own sense I was a very just unmeet person for so weighty a place . . .' The crowning glory of his mayoralty was the much postponed royal visit of Charles II to the town on 4 October. Newton with aldermen and common councilmen met the king on Christ's College Piece, 'on the greensward with mats to kneel on'. The king came in his coach, and

Newton on his knees proffered him the town mace, which he touched. Newton then presented him with a gift of 120 golden pieces; and along with the aldermen kissed the king's hand. The king did not leave his coach. The procession with Newton and his peers on horseback and accompanied by kettledrums and trumpeters rode into town. At Regent Walk the university received the king, and the corporation peeled off to the town hall for dinner. The rest of Newton's mayoralty passed off without incident, and when it came to an end he told the corporation that he was sensible that they might have suffered under his management, but he had done his best.[17]

He continued as an alderman for the rest of his life; although he was briefly dismissed by James II in 1688, but restored by William of Orange a year later. His wife Sarah died in 1716; they had been married for fifty-seven years. Newton died a year later, and was buried with his wife in St Edward's church, where their black marble memorial can still be seen in the chancel, next to that of their neighbour Owen Mayfield.

John Frohock, Samuel Newton's cousin, who took his children out of Cambridge when plague entered his household, survived and became an alderman. He met an untimely death in 1715 at the Bull in Bishopsgate, London, where a candle caught his neckcloth and other clothes and he died of his burns.[18] Newton also recorded the deaths of two of the apothecaries who had remained in Cambridge during the plague: William Frisby in 1675, and Peter Dent in 1689.[19]

Timothy Caverley, the locksmith whose son Thomas died of the plague, survived, and in 1671 was recorded as providing locks, keys and staples for the acting room at Trinity College.[20]

Once the town was declared clear of the plague, the university reconvened, colleges opened their doors, and scholars returned. One of those returning to Trinity College was Isaac Newton, who arrived back from Lincolnshire ready to articulate his ideas about gravity. He took his BA shortly after returning, and was elected a Fellow of Trinity College, becoming Lucasian Professor of Mathematics shortly after. His lectures were not a success: 'few attended and fewer understood him'.[21] He was elected a Fellow of the Royal Society in 1672, and Master of the Mint in 1696 when he moved to London, where he remained until his death. Tradition has it that the lawns outside his rooms at Trinity College still bear the scars from when he emptied out his chemical experiments.[22]

The final toll was a town still in shock for at least a decade. The graves in the churchyards and the plague pits by the pest houses eventually grassed over, but empty cottages, and the grim rows of locked pest houses waiting for the next epidemic, were constant reminders of the plague. Memories of pathetic bundles sewn into sheets and placed on to the dead carts remained. Pictures of bodies thrown into the plague pits can still send a shiver down the spine; the word 'plague' stays in the English language to describe something terrible to be avoided, and the Great Plague of 1665 and 1666 has stayed in the collective memory for three centuries.

The last serious outbreak of plague in Britain was that of 1666. Why did it disappear? The obvious answer is that the Great Fire of London destroyed insanitary and overcrowded housing and burned the thatched roofs which were the black rats' favourite environment. But the fire is now discounted as a reason for the disappearance of the plague, although it must have destroyed a whole population of plague-infected rats, and there was no great fire in Cambridge to account for the plague's absence there. However, London was an agent in the spread of infection, through blocked fleas on persons, in the straw of carriers' carts, parcels and bundles of cloth.

It is certain that the plague did not cease through medical science. This did not happen until the early twentieth century when the plague virus was identified and the ways in which it could be treated were worked out. Perhaps the virus might have disappeared due to a mutation in its form which made it less virulent. The Little Ice Age of the late seventeenth century is seen as another possible cause of the plague's disappearance, as a series of very cold winters could have killed off the virus. It is also suggested that by the end of the seventeenth century the population was better fed, and more able to withstand infection.[23]

Some authors suggest that the black rat was not the source of the plague. The argument for this goes that as the infection in England tended to arrive by sea, it could not have been brought by the black rat, as that animal prefers a quiet and cosy life, nestling in warm roofs, and is not partial to sea voyages. The black rat, therefore, must be innocent, and what was identified as bubonic plague was in fact haemorrhagic plague, which spread from person to person.[24] Nevertheless, contemporary accounts of plague victims in the seventeenth century describe the telltale buboes of bubonic plague, which was spread by rats, and when an outbreak of bubonic plague near Ipswich in 1909–11 led to the county council taking a census of rodents, colonies of black rats were found in the plague area.[25] Other suggestions are that the plague was crowded out by other virulent diseases, namely smallpox and tuberculosis.[26]

Perhaps a logical reason for the decline of the plague in England is that by the late seventeenth century a population existed that had developed an immunity to plague. In Cambridge, 384 people in 1665 and 1666 were diagnosed with plague but recovered. It is probable that they were misdiagnosed and suffered from infections such as shingles or measles; or glandular fever, which produces swellings under the arms and a high fever, while the initial stages of plague were similar to influenza, so that snap diagnoses by untrained searchers could have resulted in this being called the plague. However, prior to 1665, Cambridge experienced plague outbreaks in nearly every decade, with especially bad episodes in the early 1630s and 1640s. A population could have built up that had immunity, or anti-bodies against the plague.[27] This would have happened if victims of the plague in the 1630s and 1640s had also recovered and gone on to lead a normal life. Unfortunately, we do not know the names of those who were diagnosed with plague and recovered. However, immunity may be embedded in genes. The gene CCR5 ^32 is caused by a historically cataclysmic event, such as catching the plague and surviving.[28] If you possess this gene you may have an ancestor who caught and survived the Black Death or the Great Plague.

Plague is still endemic in rodent populations in New Mexico, South America, China, Vietnam and the Indian subcontinent. Even with modern medicine it is a horrifying disease, exhibiting the buboes described in the past, blood-clotting and the closing down of organs, swollen limbs and face, septicaemia, and gangrene in the extremities. The word still strikes fear into the heart of modern people, and, with air travel across the world the norm, is something to fear.[29] The reaction of individuals and authorities is depressingly similar to that exhibited in the seventeenth century – panic.

Appendix

How has the story of the people in this book been assembled? The first task was to identify the 1665 and 1666 plague victims, and these were found in the parish registers, which recorded the marriages, baptisms and burials of parishioners. Cambridge had fourteen parishes in the seventeenth century, each with its own register. Burials of plague victims were usually marked in the register with a black cross, the word plague or pestilence, and in one case with 'the visitation began here'. Even if plague deaths were not distinguished, clusters of deaths day after day in the same family make it obvious that these were plague deaths. Over seven hundred plague victims have been identified in Cambridge for 1665–66, but medical diagnosis was still in its infancy, and not all burials marked as plague deaths would have been from the plague. This is especially true of babies buried as plague victims, who may had died from infantile diseases as yet unknown to the seventeenth-century physician.

Parish registers come with their own problems. Parish clerks, who kept the registers, were busy men who might forget to record an event. Many entries were kept on scraps of parchment or paper before being entered in the register, and there are often gaps. The Cambridge registers for the 1640s and 1650s are incomplete with one exception, that of the outlying parish of St Andrew the Less, which has no gaps in the burial registers for 1665 and 1666. The parish clerks stayed at their posts, faithfully recording the mayhem around them, while other men fled the town.

Once the plague victims were identified their relationships and ages had to be traced through record linking. Here social custom played a part. If the couple came from different parishes it was customary for them to marry in the bride's parish, but reside in the groom's. It was also customary for the first child to be baptised in the mother's parish, so that the missing baptismal record for a child whose mother came from another parish may be found in the mother's home parish records. It is possible to trace these events in other parishes, but only with great care and the existence of other evidence pointing to the fact that this is a plague victim's family.

Parish register convention meant that a child under the age of 16 was recognised in the register as the son or daughter of X, so that even if the baptism cannot be traced it is clear that the victim was a minor. For other victims for whom there is no trace of a baptism, or other members of the family in the parish, the victim was alone. However, Cambridge was a busy market town offering trades, services and entertainment to the countryside around, and the colleges also offered employment to men and women. Many of the victims without any other identification were most likely to have been incomers to the town, lured by the prospect of employment.

Once the plague victims and their families were identified it was necessary to find out whereabouts in a parish they had lived. College, university and corporation lease books helped to compile a list of leaseholders for the period. Few people owned their own dwellings in the seventeenth century, but from the lease books emerged a number of property tycoons who were taking on leases from all three institutions and subletting and subdividing the tenements they were leasing to others. A national source, the Hearth Tax played a part in indicating the size of the house where a plague victim lived, and the Hearth Tax supplemented by probate inventories listed the contents of the house, and the number of floors it had. Of course, a person making a will which created a probate inventory had to have an estate worth £5 or more, so it was the wealthier members of Cambridge society who left wills, and not all wills have surviving inventories. However, examples of wills and inventories for a cross-section of Cambridge society exist for the later seventeenth century. A series of maps from the sixteenth and seventeenth centuries helped to build up a picture of the physical appearance of the town as these show individual buildings and houses.

Bills of Mortality for Cambridge can be found in the archives of the university library and Clare College. The custom of keeping these records started during the plague epidemic of 1630, when help had to be sought from the Privy Council as the population of Cambridge faced starvation due to the intransigence of local landholders who refused to sell the town food. The series of bills for 1665–66 gives a fortnightly or weekly overview of the numbers buried for each parish, divided into plague deaths and others, and includes the numbers of people admitted to the pest houses.

Governance of the town is recorded in the corporation common day books, the university vice-chancellor's archives and in the diary of Alderman Samuel Newton. The corporation day books listed those awarded the freedom and liberty of the town, and registered apprentices, which has been useful in tracing the occupations of plague victims, while Churchwardens' accounts and the Overseers of the Poor accounts, poor rate books, bastardy bonds and parish apprentice indentures move from town to parish level.

The life of the busy seventeenth-century housewife – either managing a large household such as that of Samuel Newton, or struggling to make ends meet in a small overcrowded tenement – has largely disappeared from the records, but can be reconstructed from the descriptions of meals provided for the corporation, Christmas feasts and the many cookery books and herbals which were published in the late seventeenth century. Businesswomen, usually widows or spinsters, do appear in the records, as landladies of inns or lease-holders of shops and stalls; and one enterprising woman took over the lease of a college tennis court.

No account of seventeenth-century Cambridge would be complete without mention of Stourbridge Fair. After St Bartholomew's Fair in Smithfield, this was the most important fair in England. These were the first events to be cancelled by the Privy Council when plague was identified. Samuel Pepys rode across the fairground in 1663, and Daniel Defoe left an in-depth description of its organisation, where the different stalls were situated, and of what was on sale. Details on the day to day running of the fair can be found in the corporation's day book and the university archives, and Samuel Newton describes the fair's opening ceremony by the mayor of Cambridge.

Any historian writing on Cambridge must be eternally grateful to Charles Henry Cooper, a nineteenth-century town clerk and anti-quarian who spent his leisure time reading and transcribing the university and the town's archives, and arranging the story of Cambridge into a chronological sequence year by year. The first volume in this sequence, *Annals of Cambridge*, was published in 1842, followed by those in 1845, 1852 and 1853. The annals are based on extracts from primary sources, without editorial comment by Cooper, and are an invaluable tool for the historian of Cambridge, and the most cited volumes on the town. Mention should also be made of another antiquarian, Dr William Mortlock Palmer, an early twentieth-century GP from Linton in Cambridgeshire who transcribed and printed a great number of original sources then held in the British Museum (now in the British Library), and the present National Archives Public Record's Office. These transcriptions are a very useful and time-saving tool for the research on history of Cambridge and Cambridgeshire.

Abbreviations

CA   Cambridgeshire Archives
CAS   Cambridge Antiquarian Society
CUA Cambridge University Archives
CUL   Cambridge University Library
CUP   Cambridge University Press
MUP Manchester University Press
OUP   Oxford University Press
PCAS *Proceedings of the Cambridge Antiquarian Society*

Dates

The great plague took place before England changed from the Gregorian to the Julian calendar. Many records dated the change of year from Lady Day (25 March), so that for example in a parish register the date 9 March 1641 is in modern usage 9 March 1642. All the dates in this book have been put into modern usage.

Notes

Preface

1. My thanks to Anne Edmundson for sharing this anecdote with me.
2. H. Cam, *Liberties and Communities in Medieval England*, Cambridge: CUP, 1944, ix.
3. C. French, 'Taking up the Challenge of Micro History: Social Conditions in Kingston upon Thames in the Late Nineteenth and Early Twentieth Centuries', *Local Historian*, Vol. 36, No. 1, 2006, 17.
4. J. Hatcher, *The Black Death*, London: Phoenix, 2008, xvi.
5. K. Wrightson, *Ralph Tailor's Summer: A Scrivener, his City and the Plague*, New Haven, CT, and London: Yale University Press, 2011.

1 The Black Horse of the Apocalypse and its Pale Rider

1. CA P22/1/1 Holy Trinity Parish Register.
2. P. Ziegler, *The Black Death*, London: Penguin, 1984, 173, 177, 178. For a detailed account of the Black Death in an East Anglian village, see J. Hatcher, *The Black Death*, London: Phoenix, 2008.
3. A.M. Campbell, *The Black Death and Men of Learning*, New York: Columbia University Press, 1931, 151.
4. C. Creighton, *A History of Epidemics in Britain*, London: Frank Cass, 1965, Vol. 1, 199, 664.
5. C.H. Cooper, *Annals of Cambridge*, Vol. III, Cambridge: W. Warwick , 1852, 180, 181.
6. *The Works of John Milton*, Ware: The Wordsworth Poetry Library, 1994, 19. The poem describes him travelling between Cambridge and the Bull, the latter being the inn in London where Cambridge carriers lodged.
7. The MS of Samuel Newton's diary is Downing College, Bowtell MS 13. This was transcribed and published by J.E. Foster. A comparison of the original with the transcript shows the transcript to be an accurate reproduction of the original, so in the interests of conservation this is the version used here. J.E. Foster ed., *The Diary of*

Samuel Newton, Alderman of Cambridge (1662–1717), Cambridge: Cambridge Antiquarian Society, 1890, vii, 16.

8. CUL UA 54/7, 11, 104, 106, 118.
9. CUL UA 54/98, 132, 204, 209.
10. N. Hodges, *Loimologia or an Historical Account of the Plague in London*, 1665, translated from the Latin in 1724. *Loimos* was the ancient Greek word for plague.
11. S. Hutton, ed., *The Conway Letters*, rev. edn, Oxford: Clarendon Press, 1992, 221–2.
12. Hodges, 4.
13. *Diary of Samuel Newton*, 12.
14. F. Herring, *Certain Rules, Directions and Advertisements for the Time of Pestilence*, 1625, facsimile edn, Theatrum Orbis Terrarum, 1973, no pagination.
15. Hodges, 62, 77.
16. W. Boghurst, *Loimographia An Account of the Great Plague of London in the Year 1665*, trans. and ed. J.L. Payne, Epidemiological Society of London, 1904, 12, 17; R. Mead, *A Discourse on the Plague*, 9th edn, 1770, 61, 65.
17. *The Pest Anatomized*, London: Wellcome Institute for the History of Medicine, 1985, 27–8.
18. L. Bradley, 'Some Medical Aspects of the Plague', in *The Plague Reconsidered*, Local Population Society, 1977, 11–24; S. Scott and C.J. Duncan, *Biology of the Plague*, Cambridge: CUP, 2007, 58.
19. Boghurst, 28.
20. College of Physicians, *Certain Directions for the Plague*, 1665, facsimile edition Theatrum Orbis Theatrum, 1975; M. Grieve, *A Modern Herbal*, Harmondsworth: Penguin, 1931 reprint 1976, 866.
21. *The Pest Anatomized*, 5, 9, 19; B. Inglis, *A History of Medicine*, Weidenfeld & Nicolson, 1965, 102–3.
22. H. Glasse, *The Art of Cookery Made Plain and Easy*, 1747, facsimile edition, London: Prospect Books, 1987, 166; Suffolk Record Office Bury, 613/1619 Barnardiston Archive Book of Recipes. Thanks to Dr Patricia Murrell for bringing this to my attention. Older readers will remember that mothballs included camphor, which has a very distinctive smell.
23. Privy Council Rules and Orders, May 1666, M. Leverett Green ed., *Calendar of State Papers Domestic, 1664–1666*, Vol. 155, No. 102, Longman, 1863.
24. CUL UA 54/78, 79/379; CA CB 1/A/8 Cambridge Corporation Common Day Book.
25. *The Pest Anatomized*, 13.

2 Fine Buildings and Bad Smells

1. E.S. DeBeer ed., *The Diary of John Evelyn*, Oxford: Clarendon Press, 2000, 236; C.H. Cooper, *Annals of Cambridge*, Vol. II, Cambridge: W. Warwick, 1852, 335.
2. St John's College Lease Book C 83/70.
3. T.D. Atkinson and J.W. Clark, *Cambridge Described and Illustrated*, 1897, 38. The stool remained there until the eighteenth century.
4. C. Morris ed., *The Illustrated Journeys of Celia Fiennes, 1685–1712*, London: Macdonald, 1982, 77–81.
5. D. Defoe, *A Tour through the Whole Island of Great Britain*, Vol. 1, first published 1724–26, new edn, London: Frank Cass 1968, 80.
6. Cooper, *Annals of Cambridge*, Vol. II, Cambridge: W. Warwick, 1852, 335.
7. CA CB 1/13/B/2 Cambridge Corporation Lease Book.
8. *Diary of John Evelyn*, 336; M. Exwood and H.G. Lehmann, trans. & eds, *The Journal of William Schellink's Travels in England 1661–1663*, Camden Society, 5th series, Vol. 1, 1993, 150.
9. CA CB/13/B/2 Cambridge Corporation Lease Book.

10. CA P26/11/1 St Botolph Overseers of the Poor Rate Book.
11. T.E. Faber, *An Intimate Picture of the Parish of St Clement's, 1250–1950*, privately published, 2006, 857.
12. Exwood and Lehmann, *Schellinks Travels in England*, 148.
13. R. Latham and W. Matthews eds, *The Diary of Samuel Pepys, Vol. 1, 1660*, London: HarperCollins, 1965, 66.
14. Cooper, *Annals of Cambridge*, Vol. III, 454, 463.
15. CUL UA T. IV.3 Letter Carriers' Licences; N. Evans and S. Rose eds, *Cambridgeshire Hearth Tax Returns*, London: The British Record Society, 2000, 20, 27, 36.
16. J.P.C. Roach ed., *The Victoria History of the Counties of England, Cambridgeshire*, London: Institute of Historical Research, Vol. II, 1967, 114.
17. CA CB 1/A/8 Cambridge Corporation Common Day Book.
18. Cooper, *Annals of Cambridge*, Vol. II, 336; Atkinson and Clark, 264; Richard Lyne, *Map of Cambridge, 1574*.
19. Atkinson and Clark, 61; J.W. Clark and A. Gray, *Old Plans of Cambridge, 1574 to 1798*, Cambridge: Bowes & Bowes, 1921, xxv.
20. Richard Lyne, *Map of Cambridge*, 1574; John Hammond, *Map of Cambridge*, 1610; John Speed, *Map of Cambridge*, 1610, David Loggan, *Map of Cambridge*, 1688, facsimiles, Cambridgeshire Records Society, 2002; Atkinson and Clark, 63.
21. Atkinson and Clark, 66–7.
22. J. Foster ed., *The Diary of Samuel Newton, Alderman of Cambridge (1662–1717)*, Cambridge: Cambridge Antiquarian Society, 1890, 4.
23. G.J. Gray, 'The Shops at the West End of Great St Mary's', *PCAS*, Vol. XIII, 1909, 241–3.
24. Atkinson and Clark, 66–7.
25. CUL UA 37/2/109.
26. Evans and Rose eds, *Hearth Tax*, 22; *Diary of Samuel Newton*, 17.
27. CA CB 1/13/B/2 Corporation Lease Book.
28. Faber, 857–82.
29. St Catharine's College Archives, Lease Book 1; Jesus College Archives, Lease Book; St John's College Archives, Lease Book C, 8; Corpus Christi Archives, CC09/181; CA CB 1/B/2 Corporation Lease Book; Downing College Library and Archives, Bowtell Ms 7.15 ; Atkinson and Clark, 72, 74, 75.
30. R. Latham and W. Matthews eds, *The Diary of Samuel Pepys, Vol. VIII, 1667*, G. Bell, 1965, 78.
31. M. Misson, *Memoirs and Observations on his travels in England*, translated in 1719, quoted in J.C. Drummond and A. Wilbraham, *The Englishman's Food*, London: Jonathan Cape, 1972, 105.
32. *Diary of John Evelyn*, 87; *Pepys, Vol. II, 1662*, 188.
33. *Diary of Samuel Newton*, 13.
34. *Diary of John Evelyn*, see n. 8. 240; *Journeys of Celia Fiennes*, 81.
35. V. Morgan, *A History of the University of Cambridge*, Vol. II, Cambridge: CUP, 2004, 222.
36. Evans and Rose eds, *Hearth Tax*, 1.
37. P. Linehan ed., *St John's College, Cambridge: A History*, Woodbridge: The Boydell Press, 2011, 126; R. Iliffe ed., *Early Biographies of Isaac Newton*, London: Pickering & Chatto, 2006, Newton's Account Book, 25.
38. CUL UA VCCt Ins I–W.
39. Cooper, *Annuals of Cambridge*, Vol. II, 335.
40. W.M. Palmer, 'The Reformation of the Corporation of Cambridge, July 1662', *PCAS*, 1912–13, 75–136.
41. *Diary of Samuel Newton*, 48.
42. CUL UA Comm. Ct 33, 37, 40, 44.
43. *Diary of Samuel Newton*, 2.

44. CA Will Register 11:30.
45. Defoe, 80.
46. Ibid., 84.
47. Descartes' Book of Colours used by Newton was probably a pirated extract from Descartes' Theory of Meteorology from Principles of Population Part IV. For further information see 5th International Conference on the History of Science, Athens, 1–3 November 2012. 'The Role of Experimentation in Descartes'. See also The Newton Project http://www.newtonproject.sussex.ac.uk page2; Illiffe ed., *Early Biographies of Isaac Newton*, John Conduit Memoir, 163, 173 Papers 43,113.
48. CUL UA Comm. Ct V.1.
49. CUL UA Comm. Ct V.12.

3 Town and Gown

1. N. Evans and S. Rose, eds, *Cambridgeshire Hearth Tax Returns*, The British Record Society, 2000, 17; CA CB 1/B/2 Cambridge Corporation Lease Book; Downing College Library and Archives, Bowtell Ms 7.13; Peterhouse Archives Lease Book 11; CUL UA D.VI.7; Jesus College Archives, Lease Book; St John's College Archives, Lease Book C.
2. Jesus College Archives, Lease Book.
3. JE. Foster ed., *The Diary of Samuel Newton, Alderman of Cambridge (1662–1717)*, Cambridge: Cambridge Antiquarian Society, 1890.
4. *Diary of Samuel Newton*, vii. The anonymous author of the entry for Samuel Newton in the *Oxford Dictionary of National Biography* gives the date as 1629 and claims that Samuel was baptised in Little St Mary's Church, but there is no evidence that this is the same Samuel Newton. Foster and the *ODNB* claim his father was a painter, but do not make it clear if this was a house painter or an artist. However, it is more likely that his father was the John Newton printer who was buried in St Edward's church in 1644, as St Edward's was the Newtons' home parish.
5. *Dairy of Samuel Newton*, 1. Although the diary proper starts in 1662 Newton kept notes from 1660, and these loose sheets were, at some point, sewn into the diary.
6. *Diary of Samuel Newton*, 2.
7. CA P 28/1/1 St Edward.
8. *Diary of Samuel Newton*, 11; Evans and Rose eds, *Hearth Tax*, 17,19.
9. *Diary of Samuel Newton*, 3; CA Will Register 11:30.
10. *Diary of Samuel Newton*, 28–30.
11. C. Willett and P. Cunningham, *Handbook of English Costume in the Seventeenth Century*, London: Faber and Faber, 1955, 159, 170, 179, 189.
12. J.C. Drummond and A. Wilbraham, *The Englishman's Food*, London: Jonathan Cape, 1959, 106.
13. H. Glasse, *The Art of Cookery Made Plain and Easy*, 1743, facsimile edn, London: Prospect Books, 1987 9; R. Price, *The Compleat Cook*, 1681, ed. M. Masson, London: Routledge, 1974, 314; lye was a mixture of ashes and salt rendered down with fat.
14. *Diary of Samuel Newton*, 11.
15. Ibid., 66.
16. Glasse, 11, 98, 99, 101, 105.
17. CA P 37/1/1 St Michael's Parish Register; CA Will Register 10:68; Evans and Rose eds, *Hearth Tax*, 29.
18. CA P 15/11/1 St Botolph Overseers of the Poor Rate Book, CA P 20/1/2 All Saints.
19. CUL UA VCCt Ins A–H, I–W; CUL UA VCCt Will Register IV; V. Morgan, *A History of the University of Cambridge*, Vol. II, Cambridge: CUP, 2006, 40–6.
20. CUL UA VCCt Ins A–H, I–W; A. Attwater, *A History of Pembroke College, Cambridge*, Cambridge: CUP, 1936, 75.

21. CUL UA VCCt Ins A–H, I–W.
22. CUL UA VCCt Ins A–H.
23. P., Linehan ed., *St John's College, Cambridge: A History*, Woodbridge: The Boydell Press, 2011, 137.
24. Ibid., 122.
25. R. Illiffe ed., *Early Biographies of Isaac Newton*, Pickering & Chatto, 2006, John Conduit Papers, 98.
26. John Conduit was married to Sir Isaac Newton's niece and collected reminiscences from Newton in old age, and letter and documents with the aim of writing a biography of the great man. This collection is in the archives of King's College Cambridge, but as well as a printed version in Illiffe, ed., *Early Biographies of Isaac Newton*, can also be accessed online at the Newton Project, http://www.newtonproject.sussex.ac.uk.
27. Illiffe ed., *Early Biographies of Isaac Newton*, Conduit Papers 77, 312, Fitzwilliam Notebook, 9.
28. Linehan, 109.
29. Evans and Rose eds, *Hearth Tax*, 35; CUL UA VCCt Ins A–H.
30. Linehan, 124.
31. CUL UA VCCt Ins A–H.
32. CUL UA VCCt Ins A–H.
33. CUL UA VCCt Will Register IV; CUL UA VCCt Ins A–H; Linehan, 123; Peterhouse Lease Book 1645–65 ff. 24, 29, 194, 226; Evans and Rose eds, *Hearth Tax*, 25.
34. CUA UA VCCt Will Register IV; CUA VCCt Ins A–H; Evans and Rose eds, *Hearth Tax*, 25.
35. CUL UA VCCt Ins A–H.
36. CUL UA VCCt 13.
37. Peterhouse Lease Book 1.11 F 61; CUL UA VCCt V. 15 Ins A–H.
38. CUL UA VCCt Ins A–H; CUL UA VCCt Wills Register IV.
39. CUL UA VCCt Ins I–W.
40. V. Morgan, *A History of the University of Cambridge*, Vol. II, Cambridge: CUP, 2004, 318; Linehan, 125.
41. Iliffe ed., *Early Biographies of Isaac Newton*, Newton's Account Book, 1, 3, 4, 9, 10.
42. R. Wroth, 'Servants at St John's College, Cambridge', unpublished Advanced Diploma Dissertation, University of Cambridge, Institute of Continuing Education, 1998.

4 Impending Disaster

1. R. Latham and A. Matthews eds, *The Diary of Samuel Pepys, 1660–1666*, Vol. VI, G. Bell, 1965, 27.
2. A. Macfarlane ed., *The Diary of Ralph Josselin, 1616–1683*, London: The British Academy, 1976, 515.
3. JE. Foster ed., *The Diary of Samuel Newton, Alderman of Cambridge (1662–1717)*, Cambridge: Cambridge Antiquarian Society, 1890, 8.
4. Nicholas Culpeper, *Culpeper's Complete Herbal* (1656), modern edn, W. Foulsham, n.d., 46, 143, 201, 206.
5. G. Hatfield, *Country Remedies*, Woodbridge: The Boydell Press, 2009, 26–7.
6. Culpeper, 219, 266.
7. *Diary of Samuel Newton*, 9.
8. Ibid., 11.
9. Ibid., 8–9.
10. Ibid., 11; R. Bird ed., *Concise Law Dictionary*, London: Sweet & Maxwell, 7th edn, 1983, 43.
11. *Diary of Samuel Newton*, 10, 11.
12. Ibid., 11.

13. *Pepys*, Vol. VI, 40.
14. *Diary of Samuel Newton*, 11.
15. Ibid., 12.
16. CA P28/1/1/ St Edward; CA Will Register 10:317.
17. M. Leverett Green ed., *Calendar of State Papers Domestic, 1664–1665*, London: Longman, 1863, 304.
18. *Diary of Samuel Newton*, 12–13.
19. J.R. Jones, *The Anglo-Dutch Wars of the Seventeenth Century*, London: Longman, 1996, 158; C. Knighton, *Pepys and the Navy*, Stroud: Sutton, 2001, 67–8.
20. A.W. Sloan, *English Medicine in the Seventeenth Century*, Durham, NC: Durham Academic Press, 1996; *Diary of Ralph Josselin*, 518.
21. V. Fumagelli, *Landscapes of Fear*, trans. S. Mitchell, Cambridge: Polity Press, 1994, 17.
22. F. Herring, *Certain Rules, Directions or Advertisements for this Time of Pestilence*, facsimile edn, Theatrum Orbis Terrarum, 1973, no pagination; B. Pullen, 'Plague and Perceptions of the Poor in Early Modern Italy', in T. Ranger and P. Slack eds, *Epidemics and Ideas*, Cambridge: CUP, 1992, 113.
23. N. Evans and S. Rose eds, *Cambridgeshire Hearth Tax Returns*, London: The British Record Society, 2000, lxxii, lxxiv, lxxix.
24. CUL UA T.IV.3.
25. *Pepys*, Vol. VI, 133; N.J. Hardy ed., *Notes and Extracts from the Hertfordshire Sessions Rolls*, Hertford: Hertfordshire County Council, Vol. I, 1909, 172.
26. W. Boghurst, *Loimographia: An Account of the Great Plague of London in the Year 1665*, trans. and ed. J.F. Payne, London: Epidemiological Society of London, 1904, 26.
27. CA P 22/1/1 Holy Trinity; CA P 20/1/2 All Saints. It is possible that these children died of measles, but they were treated as plague victims.
28. These provisions were specified in the Cambridge Plague Orders, printed in 1625, CUL UAI CUR 54/7.
29. CA P 22/1/1 Holy Trinity.
30. These incidents are taken from nineteenth-century accounts given by girls taken to the Female Refuge in East Road, Cambridge. The university proctors disturbed a couple under a market stall, but in this case the girl turned out to be only 13 years old.
31. CA P 22/1/1 Holy Trinity.
32. Evans and Rose eds, *Hearth Tax*, 2–5; CUR UIA 5417.
33. CA P 22/1/1 Holy Trinity.
34. The in-filling of this space can be seen clearly in successive maps Richard Lyne, *Map of Cambridge, 1574*; John Hammond, *Map of Cambridge, 1592*; David Loggan, *Map of Cambridge, 1688*; Evans and Rose eds, *Hearth Tax*, 2. The Lawrences' cottage stood roughly where W.H. Smith's is today.
35. CA CB 1/13/2 Cambridge Corporation Lease Book B; Evans and Rose eds, *Hearth Tax*, 2.
36. CA P 22/1/1 Holy Trinity.
37. CUL UAI CUR 54/7.
38. CA P 22/1/1 Holy Trinity.
39. A. Gray and F. Britten, *A History of Jesus College, Cambridge*, London: Heinemann, 1979, 95.
40. V. Morgan, *A History of the University of Cambridge*, Vol. II, Cambridge: CUP, 2004, 222.
41. Letter quoted in C. Creighton, *A History of Epidemics in Britain*, London: Frank Cass, 1965, Vol. I, 682.
42. CA P 23/1/1/ St Andrew the Great Parish Register; CUL UA VCCt Wills Register IV.
43. CUL UA VCCt Ins A–H.
44. R. Illiffe ed., *Early Biographies of Isaac Newton*, Pickering & Chatto, 2006, John Conduit Papers, 90.

5 The Infected Summer

1. CA CB 1/A/8 Cambridge Corporation Common Day Book, f. 199; St John's College Archives, Lease Book C 8/44, 70, 71, 475, 737; T.E. Faber, *An Intimate History of the Parish of St Clements*, Cambridge, privately printed 2006, 23, 169, 210, 857–60.
2. CA P 27/1/2 St Clement; CA P 27/14/1 St Clement Apprenticeship Indentures.
3. Matching days to historical dates can be done with C.R. Cheney, *A Handbook of Dates for Students of History*, London: Royal Historical Society, 1978, days for 1665 are on page 93.
4. CA P 27/1/2 St Clement.
5. Thomas son of David Bowen, baptised 1 March 1646, CA P 27/1/2 St Clement.
6. There is no will or probate inventory for Francis King; this account is based on several inventories taken in houses with two hearths as listed for King in the Hearth Tax, and from modest tradesmen with occupations similar to King.
7. St John's College Archives, Lease Book C 8/800; Nicholas Culpeper, *Culpeper's Complete Herbal* (1656), modern edn, W. Foulsham, n.d., 56–7.
8. M. Grieve, *A Modern Herbal*, Harmondsworth: Penguin Books, 1976, 120, quoting from Francis Bacon and John Evelyn.
9. CUL UA VCCt Wills Register IV.
10. Description of the early onset of plague is taken from N. Hodges, *Loimologia or an Historical Account of the Plague in London, 1665*, trans. from the Latin, London, 1724, 91.
11. CUL UA CUR 54/7.
12. At least two versions of the Cambridge Bills of Mortality for 1665 to 1666 have survived. One version is in the University Archives CUL UA T.X. 21 and the other is in Clare College Archives, Safe C2.27.
13. J.E. Foster ed., *The Diary of Samuel Newton, Alderman of Cambridge (1662–1717)*, Cambridge: Cambridge Antiquarian Society, 1890, 14.
14. CA CB 1/A/8 Cambridge Corporation Common Day Book.
15. S. Scott and C.J. Duncan, *The Biology of the Plague*, Cambridge: CUP, 2007, 67, 128.
16. CA P 27/1/2 St Clement.
17. CA P 27/1/2 St Clement.
18. CUL UA CUR 54/7.
19. W.G. Bell, *The Great Plague in London, 1665–1666*, London: The Bodley Head, rev. edn, 1951, 138.
20. R. Latham and W. Matthews eds, *The Diary of Samuel Pepys, 1660–1666* (1665), G. Bell, 1965, Vol. VI, 189, 201.
21. Clare College Archives, Safe C2.27.
22. CA P 23/1/1/ St Andrew the Great; CA CB 1/13/B/2 Cambridge Corporation Lease Book B; N. Evans and S. Rose eds, *Cambridgeshire Hearth Tax Returns*, London: The British Record Society, 2000, 15; CA CB 1/A/8 Cambridge Corporation Common Day Book, 128, 129.
23. CA 1/13/B/2 Cambridge Corporation Lease Book B; Evans and Rose eds, *Hearth Tax*, 5, 6; CA 1/A/8 Cambridge Corporation Common Day Book; *Diary of Samuel Newton*, 22.
24. CA P 33/1/1 St Peter; the Hearth Tax entries multiplied by 4.5 to get total number, which is 340.
25. CA P 29/1/2 St Giles; Evans and Rose eds, *Hearth Tax*, 9.
26. CA P 29/1/2 St Giles; Evans and Rose eds, *Hearth Tax*, 9.
27. Faber, 835; CA 1/A/8 Cambridge Corporation Common Day Book; *Diary of Samuel Newton*, 93.
28. St John's College Archives, Lease Book C 8/273; CA P 27/1/2 St Clement.
29. CA P 27/1/2 St Clement; CA P 25/12/4 St Benet Bastardy Bonds.
30. St John's College Archives, Lease Book C 8/273.
31. CA P 27/1/2 St Clement.

32. This argument is put forward by Lawrence Stone in *Past and Present Revisited*, London: Routledge & Kegan Paul, 1987, 314–15 and *The Family, Sex and Marriage in England 1500–1800*, Harmondsworth: Penguin, 1979. There is little evidence to support this view. Stone argues that changes in attitudes came about in the eighteenth century when children began to be recognised as individuals.
33. F. Mount, *The Subversive Family*, London: Unwin, 1982, 8, 10.
34. Quoted ibid., 115.
35. A. Macfarlane ed., *The Diary of Ralph Josselin, 1616–1683*, London: The British Academy, 1976, 201; M. Carter ed., *Mrs Elizabeth Freke Her Diary 1617–1714*, London: 1914, 200.
36. CA P 20/1/2 All Saints; CA P 22/1/1 Holy Trinity; CA P 27/1/2 St Clement.
37. Evidence from several hundred wills written by the residents of March, Cambridgeshire in the sixteenth and seventeenth centuries, and published in E. Lord, 'Reading the Will', Cambridgeshire Local History Forum, *Review*, No. 21, 2012, 16–25.

6 Falling Leaves and Sable Skies

1. J.E. Foster ed., *The Diary of Samuel Newton, Alderman of Cambridge (1662–1717)*, Cambridge Antiquarian Society, 1890, 29.
2. Ibid., 4–5.
3. Ibid., 32.
4. Ibid., 5–6.
5. CA P 21/1/1 Holy Sepulchre; CA P 21/1/11 Holy Sepulchre Overseers of the Poor Accounts.
6. CA CB 1/A/8 Cambridge Corporation Common Day Book; N. Evans and S. Rose eds, *Cambridgeshire Hearth Tax Returns*, London: The British Record Society, 2000, 12; *Diary of Samuel Newton*, 11, 26; Downing College Library and Archives, Bowtell Ms 7; CA CB 1/13/B/2 Cambridge Corporation Lease Book B.
7. CA CB 1/13/B/2 Cambridge Corporation Lease Book B.
8. J. Thirsk, *Food in Early Modern England*, Basingstoke: Hambledon Continuum, 2007, 265–70; *Diary of Samuel Newton*, 78.
9. CA P 27/1/2/ St Clement.
10. CA CB 1/A/8 Cambridge Corporation Common Day Book; CA CB 1/13/B/2 Cambridge Corporation Lease Book B; CUL UA Comm. Ct V. 13.
11. St John's College Archives Lease Book C 8; CA P 21/1/1 Holy Sepulchre.
12. Quoted in C. Creighton, *A History of Epidemics in Britain*, London: Frank Cass, 1965, Vol. I, 682.
13. CA CB 1/13/B/2 Cambridge Corporation Lease Book B; CA P 23/1/1 St Andrew the Great.
14. CA P 33/1/1 St Peter; CA P 23/1/1/ St Andrew the Great; CUL UA VCCt Wills Register IV; CUL UA VCCt Ins A–H; Evans and Rose eds, *Hearth Tax*, 24. The small amount left to Edward Bunchley probably means that arrangements for his inheritance had already been made. It was often the custom for the eldest child to be baptised in the mother's home parish; the absence of William from the will suggests an infant death.
15. T.E. Faber, *An Intimate Picture of the Parish of St Clements, 1250–1950*, Cambridge: Privately printed, 2006 ,858; CUL UA Comm. Ct V 13; *Diary of Samuel Newton*, 2, 26; CA P 27/1/2 St Clement.
16. CA P 27/1/2 St Clement.
17. CA P 37/1/1 Barton.
18. Letter from John Sturgeon to Sir Robert Harley, quoted in W. Bell, *The Great Plague of London, 1665–1666*, London: The Bodley Head, rev. edn, 1951, 30.
19. CA P 27/1/2 St Clement; St John's College Archives, Lease Book C8/737.
20. CA P 27/1/2 St Clement.

21. Faber, 210; CA Will Register 10:85.
22. Faber, 102; CA P 27/1/2 St Clement.
23. St John's College Archives Lease Book C 8/273, 367, 386; Faber, 846.
24. The list comes from the 1637 inventory of the shop goods of a Stockport haberdasher, John Bowland in C.B. Phillips and Smith eds, *Stockport Probate Records 1620–1650*, Lancashire & Cheshire Record Society, Vol. CXXXI, 1992, 220–1. No similar inventory has been traced for seventeenth-century Cambridge.
25. M. Bailey, *A Marginal Economy? East Anglian Breckland in the Middle Ages*, Cambridge: CUP, 1989. The last rabbit fur factory in Mildenhall in the Breckland did not close until the mid-twentieth century, when rabbit fur went out of fashion.
26. CA CB 1/A/8 Lease Book B. Cambridge Corporation records that William Bullin's son, another William, was apprenticed to his father, a hat dyer.
27. M. Grieve, *A Modern Herbal*, Harmondsworth: Penguin, 1976, 129, 504, 505, 597, 852.
28. Evans and Rose eds, *Hearth Tax*, 10; CA P 27/1/2 St Clement.
29. Evans and Rose eds, *Hearth Tax*, 12.
30. This description of the brazier's craft and workshop comes from J. Stow, *Description of London* (1602), ed. C. Kingsland, 1908, Vol. I, 288.
31. Hiccoughs and nose bleeds were early symptoms of the plague, Creighton, 678.
32. CA P 21/1/1 Holy Sepulchre.
33. R. Latham and W. Matthews eds, *The Diary of Samuel Pepys, 1660–1666* (1665), G. Bell, 1965, Vol. VI, 320, 328, 335.
34. Evans and Rose eds, *Hearth Tax*, 10.
35. CA P 27/1/2 St Clement.
36. Clare College Archives, Safe C2.27; CA P 33/1/1 St Peter; CA P 27/1/2 St Clement; CA P 20/1/2 All Saints; CA P 30/1/1 Great St Mary; CA P 21/1/1 Holy Sepulchre; CA P 22/1/1 Holy Trinity; CA P 23/1/1 St Andrew the Great; CA P 29/1/2 St Giles.
37. N. Hodges, *Loimologia or an Historical Account of the Plague in London* (1665), trans., London: 1724, 7–9, 11, 16.
38. W. Boghurst, *Loimographia: An Account of the Great Plague in London in the Year 1665*, trans. and ed. J.F. Payne, London: Epidemiological Society of London, 1904, 25.
39. Bell, 115.
40. CUL CUR 54.2.
41. *Pepys*, 337.

7 A Rash of Red Crosses

1. J.E. Foster ed., *The Diary of Samuel Newton, Alderman of Cambridge (1662–1717)*, Cambridge: Cambridge Antiquarian Society, 1890, 38.
2. M. Storey ed., *Two East Anglian Diaries*, Suffolk Record Society, Vol. XXXVI, 1992; J. Latham and W. Matthews eds, *The Diary of Samuel Pepys Vol. I*, 1667, HarperCollins, 1995, 322; *Pepys*, Vol. II, 1661, 238; *Pepys*, Vol. III, 1663, G. Bell, 1965, 292.
3. R. Hutton, *The Stations of the Sun*, Oxford: OUP, 1997, 31; *Diary of Samuel Newton*, 8.
4. *Dairy of Samuel Newton*, 15.
5. N. Evans and S. Rose eds, *Cambridgeshire Hearth Tax Returns*, London: The British Record Society, 2000, 7; CA P 21/1/1 Holy Sepulchre; CA CB 1/A/8 Cambridge Corporation Common Day Book; Downing College Library and Archives, Bowtell Ms 7.13; CA Will Register 10:96; CA P 29/1/2 St Giles.
6. *Pepys*, Vol. VI, HarperCollins, 1995, 338.
7. M. Leverett Green ed., *Calendar of State Papers Domestic, 1664–1666*, London: Longman, 1863, 216, 225.
8. Clare College Archives, Safe C2.27. In 1666 the Cambridge Bills of Mortality began to appear weekly rather than fortnightly. The parish registers of St Andrew the Less or Barnwell do not record any burials for 1665 or 1666. This may be because plague deaths

were never recorded or, as happened in other parishes, because the pages were torn out and destroyed, as though the inhabitants no longer wanted evidence of the dire times of 1665 and 1666.

9. CA P 27/1/2 St Clement.
10. Quoted in C.H. Cooper, *Annals of Cambridge*, Cambridge, W. Warwick, 1842–8, Vol. III, 518.
11. S. Hutton ed., *The Conway Letters*, Oxford: Clarendon Press, rev. edn, 1992, 39, 40, 46, 47, 100, 103, 104.
12. Ibid., 245–7.
13. Ibid., 248.
14. R. Spalding, ed., *The Diary of Bulstrode Whitelock, 1605–1675*, The British Academy, 1990, 703–5. Whitelock employed a 'stroker' to cure his children's ailments.
15. A. Macfarlane ed., *The Diary of Ralph Josselin, 1616–1683*, London: The British Academy, 1976, 524. Josselin lived in Earl's Colne in Essex.
16. *Calendar of State Papers Domestic, 1664–1666*, 412.
17. *Pepys*, Vol. VII, 1666, G. Bell & Son, 1965, 7.
18. E. DeBeer ed., *The Diary of John Evelyn*, Vol. III, Oxford: Clarendon Press, 2000, 437.
19. P.C. Roger, *The Dutch in the Medway*, Oxford: OUP, 1970 46, 49, 52; *Calendar of State Papers Domestic, 1664–1666*, 513.
20. Richard Lyne, *Map of Cambridge, 1574*; David Loggan, *Map of Cambridge, 1688*.
21. Evans and Rose eds, *Hearth Tax*, 33.
22. CA P 26/11/1 St Botolph, Overseers of the Poor Rate Book.
23. CA P 26/1/1 St Botolph Parish Register; CA P 26/11/1 St Botolph Overseers of the Poor Rate Book.
24. CA P 23/1/1 St Andrew the Great; Evans and Rose eds, *Hearth Tax*, 23, 27.
25. CA CB 1/13/B/2 Cambridge Corporation Lease Book B; CUL CUR 54/7.
26. R. Milward, *A Glossary of Household, Farming and Trade Terms from Probate Inventories*, Derbyshire Archaeological Society, Occasional Paper 1, 1977, 41; CUL UA VCCt Ins A–H; many parish apprentices from Cambridge were sent to Colchester to learn, for example, weaving, see CA P 24/1/1 St Benet Apprentice Indentures or CA P 24/1/1 St Andrew the Less Apprentice Indentures; CA P23/1/1 St Andrew the Great.
27. CA Will Register 10:317.
28. CA P 23/1/1 St Andrew the Great; Evans and Rose eds, *Hearth Tax*, 23.
29. CA P 23/1/1/ St Andrew the Great; Evans and Rose eds, *Hearth Tax*, 27.
30. CA P 21/1/1 Holy Trinity; CUL UA CT Comm. V.13.
31. CA P 23/1/1 St Andrew the Great; Evans and Rose eds, *Hearth Tax*, 27.
32. *Diary of Samuel Newton*, 16.
33. Evans and Rose eds, *Hearth Tax*, 213; W.K. Clay, *A History of the Parish of Waterbeach*, Cambridge: Cambridge Antiquarian Society, 1895, 22; Foster writes that Knight came from Romsey in Hampshire, but does not provide any evidence for this, *Diary of Samuel Newton*, xvi.
34. CA PCFHS 2006 An Index Translation of Waterbeach Parish Register.
35. J. Ravensdale, *The Domesday Inheritance*, London: Souvenir Press, 1986, 41.
36. W.K. Clay, *A History of the Parish of Landbeach*, Cambridge: Cambridge Antiquarian Society, 1861, 114.
37. CA P 104/1/1 Landbeach Parish Register.
38. A.P. Wright and C. Lewis eds, *The Victoria County History of the Counties of England, Cambridgeshire*, Vol. IX, London: Institute of Historical Research, 1959, 10, 32; quoted from the Landbeach Churchwardens' Accounts in Clay, 1861, 79.
39. CA P 23/1/1 St Andrew the Great; CA P 28/2/25 St Edward's Parish Apprentice Indentures no. 25.
40. G. Turner ed., *Original Letters of Early Non-conformity under Persecution and Indulgence*, Faber, 1911, 867; Hooper needed to establish a parish of legal settlement for his

children in case they needed poor relief and the evidence for this would be in the parish register; in 1666 there was no Dissenting graveyard he could use.

41. CA Bonds and Inventories 1701.
42. Clare College Archives, Safe C2.27; CA P 23/5/1 St Andrew the Great Churchwardens' Accounts; Evans and Rose eds, *Hearth Tax*, 27; CA P 23/1/1 St Andrew the Great.

8 A Harvest of Death

1. A Macfarlane, ed., *The Diary of Ralph Josselin, 1616–1685*, London: The British Academy, 1976, 528.
2. Cumulonimbus capillatus or thunderheads can contain the equivalent energy of ten atom bombs as dropped on Hiroshima. R. Hamblyn *The Cloud Book: How to Understand the Skies.* In association with the Met Office, Cincinnati, OH: David & Charles, 2008, 49–50.
3. CA P 25/1/1 St Benet's Parish Register; CA P 22/1/1 Holy Trinity; CA P 20/1/2 All Saints.
4. The Joyces appear in St Benet's Parish Register from 1629 onwards, but they do not appear in the Poor or Church Rate Books, or the Hearth Tax. Perhaps they were too poor to pay the rates, but if this was the case they should have appeared in the Hearth Tax with a note that they were exempted by poverty.
5. CA P 25/1/1 St Benet's Parish Register.
6. CUL UA Comm. Ct:V.13.
7. CA P 25/1/1 St Benet's Parish Register.
8. Clare College Archives, Safe C2.27, Cambridge Bills of Mortality 11–19 July 1666.
9. CA P 23/1/1 Holy Trinity; N. Evans and S. Rose eds, *Cambridgeshire Hearth Tax Returns*, London: The British Record Society, 2000, 4.
10. Jesus College Archives, Lease Book; Evans and Rose eds, *Hearth Tax*, 16.
11. CA P 20/1/1 All Saints.
12. Evans and Rose eds, *Hearth Tax*, 4.
13. Quoted in W.G. Bell, *The Great Plague in London, 1665–1666*, London: The Bodley Head, 1951, 96.
14. CA P 30/11/1 Great St Mary Overseers of the Poor, Poor Rate Book.
15. CA P 22/1/1 Holy Trinity; Evans and Rose eds, *Hearth Tax*, 4; CA P 22 22/5/3 Holy Trinity Overseers of the Poor Rate Book.
16. CA P St Benet Overseers of the Poor; CA P 25/1/1 St Benet Parish Register.
17. CA P 20/1/2 All Saints; Evans and Rose eds, *Hearth Tax*, 16; Royal Commission on Historical Monuments, *City of Cambridge*, London: HMSO, 1988, Vol. II, 348–9.
18. A will-maker had to have property worth £5 or over or it was not worth the diocesan court of the church granting probate, as their fine would have been negligible.
19. CA P 30/1/1 Great St Mary's; Keith Wrightson *Ralph Tailor's Summer: A Scrivener, his City and the Plague*, New Haven and London: Yale University Press, 2011 describes how the scrivener Ralph Tailor of Newcastle-upon-Tyne took down wills from plague victims as he stood outside their houses.
20. CA Will Registers 10:67, 68; CA P 30/4/2 Great St Mary Church Rate Book.
21. CUL UA VCCt Ins A–H, I–W.
22. Downing College Library and Archives, Bowtell Ms 7; Evans and Rose eds, *Hearth Tax*, 34.
23. CA Will Register 10:72.
24. CA P 22/1/1 Holy Trinity.
25. RCHM, Vol. I, lxxix, lxxxiii.
26. RCHM, Vol. II, 153, 157.
27. CA CB 1/13/B/2 Cambridge Corporation Lease Book B.
28. CUL UA Comm Ct V. 112.
29. CA P 23/1/1 St Andrew the Great.

30. CA P 27/1/2 St Clement.
31. Richard Lyne, *Map of Cambridge, 1574*; David Loggan, Map of Cambridge, 1688; T.E. Faber, *An Intimate Picture of the Parish of St Clements, 1250–1950*, Cambridge: privately printed, 2006, 55.
32. Nicholas Culpeper, *Culpeper's Complete Herbal* (1656), W. Foulsham & Son edn, n.d. 114, 115.
33. C.R. Cheney ed., *A Handbook of Dates for Students of English History*, London: Royal Historical Society, 1978, 133; E. DeBeer ed., *Diary of John Evelyn*, Vol. III, 1650–1672, Oxford: Clarendon Press, 2000, 446.
34. R. May, *The Accomplisht Cook or The Art and Mystery of Cookery*, 1685, facsimile edn, London: Prospect Books, 1994, no pagination.
35. CA P 20/1/2 All Saints; CA P 21/1/1 Holy Sepulchre; CA P 22/1/1/ Holy Trinity; CA P 30/1/1/ Great St Mary's; CA P 26/1/2 St Botolph; CA P 25/1/2 St Clement.
36. CA P 20/1/2 Great St Mary's Overseers of the Poor, Poor Rate Book; Evans and Rose eds, *Hearth Tax*, 14; *PCAS*, Vol. XIII, 1909, 235–49.
37. CA P 22/1/1 Holy Trinity.
38. CA P 28/1/1 St Edward.
39. D. Cressy, *Birth, Marriage and Death*, Oxford: OUP, 1997, 201. My aunt was probably one of the last women to be churched. This took place in or about 1938 in Outwood, Surrey. She said afterwards that she was forced into it by the vicar, and she was chapel anyway!
40. R. Latham and W. Matthews eds, *The Diary of Samuel Pepys 1660–1666*, Vol. VII, 1666, G. Bell, 1972, 262–3.
41. Corpus Christi College Archives, CCO9/60a; Evans and Rose eds, *Hearth Tax*, 24.
42. CA P 23/1/1 St Andrew the Great; Evans and Rose eds, *Hearth Tax*, 24.
43. Clare College Archives, Safe C2.27.
44. M. Everett Green ed., *Calendar of State Papers Domestic 1664–1666*, London: Longman, 1863, 17.
45. CA P 27/1/2 St Clement.
46. CA P 40/1/1 Chesterton.
47. *Diary of Ralph Josselin*, 529.
48. Peterhouse Lease Book I.II; Downing College Library and Archives, Bowtell Ms 7; CA CB 1/13/B/2 Cambridge Corporation Lease Book.
49. *Calendar of State Papers Domestic 1664–1666*, 53.
50. M. Overton, *The Agricultural Revolution in England*, Cambridge: CUP, 1996, 12.
51. P.J. Bowden ed., *Economic Change: Wages, Profits and Rents, 1500–1750*, Cambridge: CUP, 1990, 320.
52. CA CB 1/A/8 Cambridge Corporation Common Day Book.
53. Clare College Archives, Safe C2.27.
54. CA P 22/1/1 Holy Trinity; Evans and Rose eds, Hearth Tax, 4.

9 The Beginning of the End of the Pestilence

1. Samuel Pepys and John Evelyn left eye-witness accounts of the fire, describing citizens escaping with their possessions, and the attempts of the king and the duke of York to stem the flames. Pepys took his money and plate to Bethnal Green.
2. J.E. Foster ed., *The Diary of Samuel Newton, Alderman of Cambridge (1662–1717)*, Cambridge: Cambridge Antiquarian Society, 1890, 15–16.
3. The Frohock family survived as butchers into the twentieth century with a shop in Waterbeach, Cambridgeshire, and one member is listed in the 2012 telephone directory for Cambridge.
4. CA CB 1/13/B/2 Cambridge Corporation Lease Book B.
5. CA P 31/1/1 Little St Mary's.

6. N. Evans and S. Rose eds, *Cambridgeshire Hearth Tax Returns*, London: The British Record Society, 2000, 76.
7. Ibid., 35–6; CA P 32/1/1 St Michael's.
8. Royal Commission on Historical Monuments, *City of Cambridge*, London: HMSO, 1959, republished 1988, Vol. I, 117.
9. CA P 222/5/3 Holy Trinity Churchwarden Accounts.
10. R. Iliffe ed., *Early Biographies of Isaac Newton*, Pickering & Chatto, 2006, Newton's Notebook 1, 5.
11. What is not known is whether the doors of the less wealthy could be locked. Is it a myth that in the past cottage doors could be left un-locked, and neighbours could walk straight in?
12. Royal Commission on Historical Monuments, *Cambridge*, Vol. I, 119.
13. CUL UA Comm. Ct VI, 13.
14. Evans and Rose eds, *Hearth Tax*, 36; CA P 31/1/1 St Michael's.
15. Clare College Archives, Safe C2.27.
16. Iliffe ed., *Early Biographies of Isaac Newton*, 4, 10, 11.
17. CA CB 1/13/B/2 Cambridge Corporation Lease Book B; CUL UA D.VI:7; Downing College Library and Archives Bowtell Ms 7; CUL UA D.II: Evans and Rose eds, *Hearth Tax*, 21, 23.
18. CA Will Register 10:73.
19. Clare College Archives, Safe C2.27; CA KB 1/A/8 Cambridge Corporation Common Day Book.
20. CA P 30/1/1 Great St Mary's.
21. CA Will Register 10:66.
22. W.M. Palmer 'The Reformation of the Corporation of Cambridge, July 1662', *PCAS*, Vol. XI, new series, 1912–13, 34.
23. *Diary of Samuel Newton*, 42, 49, 92–3.
24. Pepys, Evelyn and Josselin all describe the unceasing rain and floods of October 1666: R. Latham and W. Matthews eds, *The Diary of Samuel Pepys, 1660–1666*. Vol. VII, 324, 325, 328; E. DeBeer ed., *Diary of John Evelyn*, Oxford: Clarendon Press, 2000 466; A. Macfarlane ed., *The Diary of Ralph Josselin, 1616–1683*, London: The British Academy, 1976, 531.
25. Clare College Archives, Safe C2.27.
26. St John's College Archives, Lease Book C 8/800; Evans and Rose eds, *Hearth Tax*, 7, 12, 21.
27. CA P 97/1/2 Impington.
28. CA P 23/1/1 St Andrew the Great.
29. *Pepys*, Vol. VII, 352; *Diary of John Evelyn*, 466; Iliffe, ed., *Early Biographies of Isaac Newton*, 11.
30. *Diary of Samuel Newton*, 16.
31. CA P 23/1/1 St Andrew the Great; CA P 22/1/1 Holy Trinity.
32. *Diary of Samuel Newton*, 16; Evans and Rose eds, *Hearth Tax*, 18.
33. Clare College Archives, Safe C2.27.
34. CA P 22/1/1 Holy Trinity; CA P 21/1/1 Holy Sepulchre.
35. *Pepys*, Vol. VII, 393; *Diary of Ralph Josselin*, 532; *Diary of Samuel Newton*, 16.
36. CA P 22/1/1 Holy Trinity; CA P 23/1/1 St Andrew the Great; CA P 29/1/2 St Giles; CA P 31/1/1 Little St Mary; Clare College Archives, Safe C2.27; CA P 30/1/1 Great St Mary's.
37. *Diary of Samuel Newton*, viii, ix, 16.
38. Clare College Archives, Safe C2.27.
39. CA CB 1/A/8 Cambridge Corporation Common Day Book; *Diary of Samuel Newton*, 18.
40. *Pepys*, Vol. VII, 426.

NOTES to pp. 128–36

10 The Final Toll

1. Clare College Archives, Safe C2.27.
2. Quoted in A. Dyer, 'The Influence of Bubonic Plagues in England, 1500–1667', *Medical History*, Vol. 22, No. 3, July 1978, 311–12.
3. Ibid., 312.
4. N. Evans and S. Rose eds, *Cambridgeshire Hearth Tax Returns*, London: The British Record Society, 2000, lxxxi–lxxxii.
5. A. Whiteman ed., *The Compton Census of 1676*, London: The British Academy, 1986, 159, 165, 167.
6. Dyer, 312.
7. CA P 22/1/1 Holy Trinity.
8. Unfortunately there is no record of the names of the Cambridge searchers and watchmen.
9. CUL UA CUR 54.2.
10. CUL UA CUR 54.2.
11. M. Power ed., *Liverpool Town Books 1649–1671*, Lancashire & Cheshire Record Society, Vol. CXXVI, 1999, 52, 83.
12. CA CB 1/A/8 Cambridge Corporation Common Day Book.
13. J. Gray, *Biographical Notes on Mayors of Cambridge*, Cambridge: Cambridge Chronicle, 1921, 40–1.
14. E. Foster ed., *The Diary of Samuel Newton, Alderman of Cambridge (1662–1717)*, Cambridge: Cambridge Antiquarian Society, 1890, 17, 23.
15. Ibid., 16–24.
16. CA P 28/1/1 St Edward; *Diary of Samuel Newton*, 42–3.
17. Ibid., 51, 63–5, 67.
18. Ibid., 93, 127.
19. Ibid., 73, 103.
20. A.H. Nelson, *Early Cambridge Theatres*, Cambridge: CUP, 1994, 58.
21. R. Iliffe ed., *Early Biographies of Isaac Newton*, Pickering & Chatto, 2006, Conduit Papers, 154.
22. Personal information from Mark Donachy, Cambridge Blue Badge Guide.
23. S. Scott and C.J. Duncan, *The Biology of the Plague. Evidence from Historical Populations*, Cambridge: CUP, 2007, 365, 383.
24. Ibid., 356, 358.
25. D. Van Zwanenberg, 'The Last Epidemic of Plague in England, 1906–1918', *Medical History*, Vol. XIV, No. 1, 1970, 63–74.
26. Scott and Duncan, 356.
27. A discussion with a public health officer who has worked in England and the Tropics suggests that immunity is the most probable answer to the disappearance of the plague from England.
28. Scott and Duncan, 358.
29. R. Henderson, 'A–Z of Modern Maladies, Yersina Pestis', *Sunday Times*, 28 February 2010; L. Marker, 'We survived the bubonic plague', *Guardian Weekend*, 6 February 2010, 12.

BIBLIOGRAPHY

Primary Sources Manuscripts

Cambridge Archives (Cambridgeshire Record Office) [CA]

Parish Registers, Cambridge

P 20/1/2 All Saints
P 30/1/1 Great St Mary's
P 21/1/1 Holy Sepulchre
P 22/1/1 Holy Trinity
P 31/1/1 Little St Mary
P 23/1/1 St Andrew the Great
P 24/1/1 St Andrew the Less
P 25/1/1 St Benedict also known as Bene't
P 26/1/2 St Botolph
P 27/1/2 St Clement
P 28/1/1 St Edward
P 29/1/2 St Giles
P 31/1/1 St Michael
P 33/1/1 St Peter

Parish Registers Cambridgeshire

P 37/1/1 Barton
P 39/1/1 Cherry Hinton
P 40/1/1 Chesterton
P 67/1/2 Ely, Holy Trinity
P 82/1/1 Haddenham
P 93/1/1 Histon
P 97/1/2 Impington

P 104/1/1 Landbeach
An Index Transcription of the Parish Register of Waterbeach, CFHS, 2006
P 170/B/1 Whittlesey St Andrew Burial Register
Wisbech An Index Transcription of the Parish Burial Register of St Peter's Wisbech, CFHS, 2008; An Indexed Transcription of the Parish Register of Waterbeach, CFHS, 2006

Cambridge Corporation Records

CB 1/A/8 Cambridge Corporation Common Day Book 1647–1681
CB 1/A/32 Cambridge Corporation Miscellanea Book C *c.* 1550–1872
CB 1/13/B/2 Cambridge Corporation Lease Book B 1638–1712

Cambridge Parish Records

P 21/1/11 Holy Sepulchre, Overseers of the Poor Accounts
P 22/5/1 Holy Trinity Churchwarden Accounts
P 23/5/1 St Andrew the Great Churchwardens' Accounts 1651–1708
P 24/11/1 St Andrew the Less Overseers of the Poor Accounts 1652
P 25/6/1 St Benedict Churchwardens' Property 1672
P 25/11/1 St Benedict Overseers of the Poor Rate Book 1653–1666
P 25/14/4/1—18 St Benedict Apprentice Inventories 1629–1820
P 25/15/4 St Benedict Bastardy Bonds 1658–1665
P 26/5/2 St Botolph Churchwardens' Accounts 1646–1715
P 26/11/1 St Botolph Overseers' of the Poor Rate Book 1660–1669
P 27/14/1 St Clement Apprenticeship Indentures 1660–1669
P 28/2/ 1–37 St Edward's Apprentice Indentures
P 29/8/3 St Giles Vestry Audit Book 1620–1807
P 30/4/2 Great St Mary Churchwardens' Accounts 1635–1699
P 30/11/1 Great St Mary Overseers of the Poor, Poor Rate Book 1648–1672
P 31/4/1 Little St Mary Churchwardens' Rate Book 1581–1843
P 33/8/3 St Peter's Vestry Audit Book 1586–1712

Bonds and Inventories, 1688, 1701
VC 31:85 Vice-Chancellor's Will Register 31:85
Will Registers 10:4–6, 8, 17, 23, 28, 43, 44, 47–52, 58–68, 72–5, 85, 96, 317; 11:30

Cambridge University Library [CUL]

UA Comm. Ct V.1 Commissary Court Archives, Papers relating to Stourbridge Fair
UA Comm. Ct V. 2–4 Commissary Court Archives, Acta at Barnwell (Midsummer) Fair
UA Comm. Ct V. 5–16, 18 Commissary Court Archives, Acta at Stourbridge Fair 1562–1855
UA Comm. Ct V. 19 Commissary Court Archives, Text confirming the University's liberties at Stourbridge Fair
UA Comm. Ct V. 112
UA CUR 4–13 University Registry Guard Book Miscellanea
UA CUR 14 University Registry Guard Book Stokys Alms Houses
UA CUR 18, 18.2 University Registry Guard Book Great St Mary's Church
UA CUR 21 University Registry Guard Book Ms Probate Inventories
UA CUR 37 University Registry Guard Book Town, 10 vols
UA CUR 54, 54.2 University Registry Guard Book Plague, 7, 11, 78, 79.379, 98, 104, 106, 118, 132, 204, 209

UA CUR 122 University Registry Guard Book Benefaction of John Crane
UA D.1.1 Deed Register Leasebook 1665–1866
UA D.V1.7 Valuations Book
UA T.1 Record relating the licensing of alehouse keepers
UA T.IV.3 Letter carriers' bonds, licences and papers
UA T.X.19 Act Book of the Court of the Vice-Chancellor and Mayor
UA T.X.20 Miscellaneous Account Book of Dr Butts 1629–1631
UA T.X.21 Cambridge Bills of Mortality 1665–1667
UA VCCt Ins A–H, I–W
UA VCCt Wills Register IV

Christ's College Archives

Lease book 1

Clare College Archives

Safe C2.27

Corpus Christi College Archives

CCO9/09/124, CC09/181, CC09/60a

Downing College Library and Archives

Bowtell Ms 7

Jesus College Archives

Peterhouse Lease Book 1.II

St Catharine's College Archives

Lease Book 1

St John's College Archives

Lease Book C

Suffolk Record Office

Bury St Edmunds Acc 613/1619

Printed Primary Sources

The Accomplisht Ladies Delight, 1677
Baggs, T. and P. Bryan eds, *Cambridge 1574–1904*, A portfolio of maps, Cambridgeshire Records Society, 2002
Boghurst, W. *Loimographia: An Account of the Great Plague in London in the Year 1665*, trans. and ed. J.L. Payne, Epidemiological Society of London, 1904
Carter, M. ed., *Mrs Elizabeth Freke Her Diary, 1617–1714*, London, 1914
College of Physicians, *Certain Directions for the Plague*, 1665, facsimile edn, Theatrum Orbis Terrarum, 1975

Cooper, C.H. *Annals of Cambridge*, Cambridge: W. Warwick, 1842–52

Cooper, T. ed., *The Journal of William Dowsing*, London: The Ecclesiological Society, 2007

The Court and Kitchen of Elizabeth, commonly called Joan Cromwell, 1664, notes by M. Liquorice, Cambridge: Cambridgeshire Libraries, 1983

Culpeper, Nicholas, *Culpeper's Complete Herbal* (1656), new edn, London: W. Foulsham, n.d.

DeBeer, E. ed., *Diary of John Evelyn*, 6 vols, Oxford: Clarendon Press, 2000

Defoe, D. *A Tour through the Whole Island of Great Britain*, London: Frank Cass, new edn, 1968

De La Bedoyre, G. ed., *The Letters of Samuel Pepys 1656–1703*, Woodbridge: The Boydell Press, 2006

Digby, K. *The Closet Opened*, ed. J. Stevens and P. Daniels, 1669 facsimile edn, Prospect Books, 1997

Evans, N. and S. Rose eds, *Cambridgeshire Hearth Tax Returns*, London: The British Record Society, 2000

Exwood, M. and H.L. Lehmann, trans. and ed., *The Journal of William Schellink's Travels in England 1661–1663*, Camden Society, 5th series, Vol. 1, 1993

Foster, J.E. ed., *The Diary of Samuel Newton, Alderman of Cambridge (1662–1717)*, Cambridge: Cambridge Antiquarian Society, 1890

The Gentleman's Kitchen, 1683

Glasse, H. *The Art of Cookery Made Plain and Easy*, 1747 facsimile edn, London: Prospect Books, 1987

Hardy, N.J. *Notes and Extracts from Hertfordshire Sessions Rolls*, Hertford: Hertfordshire County Council, 1919

Herring, R. *Certain Rules, Directions and Advertisements for the Time of Pestilence*, 1625; facsimile edn Theatrum Orbis Terrarum, 1973

Hill, R. ed., *The Correspondence of Thomas Corie, Town Clerk of Norwich 1664–1687*, Norfolk Record Society, 1956

Hodges, N. *Loimologia or an Historical Account of the Plague in London* (1665), trans., London: 1724

Hutton, S. ed., *The Conway Letters*, Oxford: Clarendon Press, rev. edn, 1992

Iliffe, R. ed., *Early Biographies of Isaac Newton*, Pickering & Chatto, 2006

Latham, R. and W. Matthews eds, *The Diary of Samuel Pepys, 1667: 1660–1662*, 11 vols, London: HarperCollins, 1995, *1663–1666*, London: G. Bell, 1965

Leverett Green, M. ed., *Calendar of State Papers Domestic, 1664–1666*, London: Longman, 1863

Macfarlane, A. ed., *The Diary of Ralph Josselin, 1616–1683*, 11 vols, London: The British Academy, 1976

May, R. *The Accomplisht Cook or The Art and Mystery of Cookery* (1685) facsimile edn, London: Prospect Books, 1994

Mead, R. *A Discourse on the Plague*, 9th edn 1770

Metters, A. ed., *The King's Lynn Port Books, 1610–1614*, Norwich: Norfolk Record Society, 2009

Morris, C. ed., *The Illustrated Journeys of Celia Fiennes 1685–1712*, London: Macdonald, 1982

Nelson, A.H. *Records of Early English Drama, Cambridgeshire*, Toronto: University of Toronto Press, 1989

Palmer, W.M. *Cambridgeshire Subsidy Rolls, 1250–1691*, Norwich: Goose, 1912

Phillips, C.B. and J. Smith eds, *Stockport Probate Records, 1620–1650*, Lancashire & Cheshire Record Society, Vol. CXXXI, 1992

Price, R. *The Complete Cook* 1681; ed. M. Masson, London: Routledge, 1974

Seaman, P., J. Pound and R. Smith eds, *Norfolk Hearth Tax Exemptions*, London: British Record Society, 2001

Spalding, R. ed., *The Diary of Bulstrode Whitelock 1605–1675*, London: The British Academy, 1990

Storey, M. ed., *Two East Anglian Diaries*, Suffolk Record Society, Vol. XXXVI, 1992

Stow, J. *Description of London*, ed. C. Kingsland, 1908

Turner, G. ed., *Original Letters of Early Non-conformity under Persecution and Indulgence*, Faber, 1911

Whiteman, A. ed., *The Compton Census of 1676*, London: The British Academy, 1986

The Works of John Milton, Ware, Hartfordshire: The Wordsworth Poetry Library, 1994

Secondary Sources: Books

Atkinson, T.D. and J.W. Clark *Cambridge Described and Illustrated*, 1897

Attwater, A. *Pembroke College, Cambridge*, Cambridge: CUP, 1936

Bailey, M. *A Marginal Economy? East Anglian Breckland in the Late Middle Ages*, Cambridge: CUP, 1989

Barry, J. ed., *The Tudor and Stuart Town, 1530–1688*, London: Longman, 1990

Bell, W. *The Great Plague in London, 1665–1666*, London: The Bodley Head, rev. edn, 1951

Bendall, S., C. Brooke and P. Collinson, *A History of Emmanuel College, Cambridge*, Woodbridge: The Boydell Press, 1999

Berg, M. *The Age of Manufacturers 1700–1820*, London: Routledge, 1994

Bird, R. ed., *Concise Law Dictionary*, London: Sweet & Maxwell, 7th edn, 1983

Bowden, P.J. *Economic Change, Wages, Profit and Rents, 1500–1750*, Cambridge: CUP, 1990

Bradley, L. *The Plague Reconsidered*, Local Population Society, 1977

Burnby, I. G. *A Study of the English Apothecary from 1666–1760*, London: Wellcome Institute for the History of Medicine, 1983

Cam, H. *Liberties and Conmunities in Medieval England*, Cambridge: CUP, 1944

Campbell, A.M. *The Black Death and Men of Learning*, New York: Columbia University Press, 1931

Cheney, C.R. ed., *A Handbook of Dates for Students of History*, London: Royal Historical Society, 1978

Cipolla, C.M. *Christofano and the Plague*, London: Collins, 1973

——, *Fighting the Plague in Seventeenth-Century Italy*, Madison: University of Wisconsin Press, 1981

Clark, J.W. and A. Gray, *Old Plans of Cambridge 1574 to 1798*, Cambridge: Bowes & Bowes, 1921

Clark, P. and P. Slack, *English Towns in Transition, 1500–1700*, Oxford: OUP, 1976

Clay, W.K. *A History of the Parish of Landbeach*, Cambridge: Cambridge Antiquarian Society, 1861

——, *A History of the Parish of Waterbeach*, Cambridge: Cambridge Antiquarian Society, 1895

Creighton, C. *A History of Epidemics in Britain*, London: Frank Cass, 1965

Cressy, D. *Birth, Marriage and Death*, Oxford: OUP, 1997

Drummond, J.C. and A. Wilbraham, *The Englishman's Food*, London: Jonathan Cape, 1972

Faber, T.E. *An Intimate Picture of the Parish of St Clements, 1250–1950*, Cambridge: privately printed, 2006

Fumagelli, V. *Landscapes of Fear*, trans. S. Mitchell, Cambridge: Polity Press, 1994

Gray, A. and F. Britton, *A History of Jesus College, Cambridge*, London: Heinemann, 1979

Gray, J. *Biographical Notes on the Mayors of Cambridge*, Cambridge: Cambridge Chronicle, 1921

Grell, O.P. and A. Cunningham, *Religious Medicine*, Aldershot: Scolar Press, 1996

Grieve, M. *A Modern Herbal*, Harmondsworth: Penguin, 1931; rep. 1976

Hainsworth, P.R. and C. Church, *The Anglo-Dutch Naval Wars 1652–1674*, Stroud: Sutton, 1998

Hamblyn, R. *The Cloud Book*, Cincinnati: David & Charles, 2008

Hatcher, J. *The Black Death*, Phoenix, 2008

Hatfield, G. *Country Remedies*, Woodbridge: The Boydell Press, 2009

Horrox, R. ed., *The Black Death*, Manchester: MUP, 1994

Hutton, R. *The Stations of the Sun*, Oxford: OUP, 1997

Inglis, B. *A History of Medicine*, London: Weidenfeld & Nicolson, 1965

Jones, J.R. *The Anglo-Dutch Wars of the Seventeenth Century*, London: Longman, 1996

Knighton, C. *Pepys and the Navy*, Stroud: Sutton, 2001

Laslett, P. *The World We Have Lost*, London: Methuen, 1979

Linehan, P. ed., *St John's College, Cambridge: A History*, Woodbridge: The Boydell Press, 2011

Lord, E. *A Road through Time*, Cambridge: EAH Press, 2013

Matthews, A.G. *Calumny Revisited*, Oxford: OUP, 1934

Meadows, P. ed., *Ely Bishops and Diocese 1109–2009*, Woodbridge: The Boydell Press, 2010

Milward, R. *A Glossary of Household, Farming and Trade Terms for Probate Inventories*, Derbyshire Archaeological Society, Occasional Paper 1, 1977

Morgan, V. *A History of the University of Cambridge*, Vol. II, Cambridge: CUP, 2004

Mount, F. *The Subversive Family*, London: Unwin Paperbacks, 1982

Nelson, A.H. *Early Cambridge Theatres*, Cambridge: CUP, 1994

Nichols, J. *The History and Antiquities of Barnwell Abbey and of Stourbridge Fair*, 1886

Overton, M. *The Agricultural Revolution in England*, Cambridge: CUP, 1996

The Pest Anatomized: Five Centuries of Plague in Western Europe, London: Wellcome Institute for the History of Medicine, 1985

Power, M. ed., *Liverpool Town Books 1649–1671*, Lancashire & Cheshire Record Society, Vol. CXXXVI, 1999

Ranger, T. and P. Slack eds, *Epidemics and Ideas*, Cambridge: CUP, 1992

Ravensdale, J., *The Domesday Inheritance*, London: Souvenir Press, 1986

Rawcliffe, C. *Medicine and Society in Later Medieval England*, Stroud: Sutton, 1995

Roach, H. *A Dictionary of English County Physicians 1603–1643*, London: Dawson, 1962

Roach, J.P.C. *The Victoria History of the Counties of England, Cambridgeshire*, Vol. III, London: Institute of Historical Research, 1967

Roger, P.C. *The Dutch in the Medway*, Oxford: OUP, 1970

Rogers, C.D. and J. Smith, *Local History in England*, Manchester: MUP, 1991

Royal Commission on Historical Monuments, *City of Cambridge*, London: HMSO, 1988

Scott, S. and C.J. Duncan, *The Biology of the Plague: Evidence from Historical Populations*, Cambridge: CUP, 2007

Slack, P. *The Impact of Plague in Tudor and Stuart England*, London: Routledge, 1985

Sloan, A.W. *English Medicine in the Seventeenth Century*, Durham, NC: Durham Academic Press, 1996

Stone, L. *The Family, Sex and Marriage in England 1500–1800*, Harmondsworth: Penguin, 1979

Thirsk, J. *Food in Early Modern England*, Basingstoke: Hambledon Continuum, 2007

Thursley, C. and D. Thursley, *Index of Probate Records of the Consistory Court of Ely 1449–1858*, London: The British Record Society, 1995

Twigg, J. *The University of Cambridge and the English Revolution*, Woodbridge: The Boydell Press, 1990

Varley, F.J. *Cambridge and the Civil War* Cambridge: W. Heffer, 1935

Walker. T. ed., *Admissions to Peterhouse, Cambridge*, Cambridge: CUP, 1912

Willet, C. and P. Cunningham, *Handbook of English Costume in the Seventeenth Century*, London: Faber and Faber, 1955

Wilson, C. *Profit and Power*, London: Longman, 1957

Wright, A.P. and Lewis C. eds, *The Victoria History of the Counties of England, Cambridgeshire*, Vol. IX, London: Institute of Historical Research, 1959

Wrightson, K. *Ralph Tailor's Summer: A Scrivener, his City and the Plague*, New Haven, CT, and London: Yale University Press, 2011

Ziegler, P. *The Black Death*, Harmondsworth: Penguin, 1984

Secondary Sources: Articles

Bradley, L. 'The Geographical Spread of the Plague', in *The Plague Reconsidered*, Local Population Society, 1977

——, 'The Most Famous of All English Plagues', in *The Plague Reconsidered*, Local Population Society, 1977

——, 'Some Medical Aspects of the Plague' in *The Plague Reconsidered*, Local Population Society, 1977

Cessford, M. 'Excavations of the Civil War Bastion Ditch of Cambridge Castle' *PCAS*, Vol. XCVII, 2008

Dyer, A. 'The Influence of Bubonic Plagues in England 1500–1667', *Medical History*, Vol. 22, No. 3, July 1978

French, C. 'Taking up "the challenge of micro-history": social conditions in Kingston upon Thames in the late nineteenth and early twentieth centuries', *Local Historians*, Vol. 36, No. 1, 2006, 17–28

Goose, N. 'Household Size and Structure in Early Stuart Cambridge', in J. Barry ed., *The Tudor and Stuart Town, 1536–1688*, London: Longman, 1990

Gray, G.J. 'The Shops at the West End of Great St Mary's', *PCAS*, Vol. XIII, 1909

Grell, O.P. 'Prayer and Physic: Helmontian Medicine in Restoration England', in O.P. Grell and A. Cunningham, *Religious Medicine*, Aldershot: Scolar Press, 1996

Henderson, R. 'A–Z of Modern Maladies, Yersinia Pestis', *Sunday Times*, 28 February 2010

King, H. 'Nathaniel Hodges', *Oxford Dictionary of National Biography*, Oxford: OUP, 2005

Lord, E. 'Reading the Will', Cambridge Local History Forum, *Review*, No. 21, 2012, 16–25

Marker, L. 'We Survived Bubonic Plague', *Guardian Weekend Section*, 6 February 2010

Palmer, W.M. 'The Reformation of the Corporation of Cambridge, July 1662', *PCAS*, Vol. VII, OS XVII, 1912–13

Pullen, B. 'Plague and Perceptions of the Poor in Early Modern Italy', in T. Ranger and P. Slack eds, *Epidemics and Ideas*, Cambridge: CUP, 1992

Slack, P. 'William Boghurst', *Oxford Dictionary of National Biography*, Vol. 6, Oxford: OUP, 2005

Stokes, H.P, 'Outside Trumpington Gate', *PCAS*, Vol. XII, 1908

Van Zwanenberg, D. 'The Last Epidemic of Plague in England, 1906–1918', *Medical History*, Vol. XIV, No. 1, 1970

Maps

Hammond, John, *Map of Cambridge, 1610*

Loggan, David, *Map of Cambridge, 1688*

Lyne, Richard, *Map of Cambridge, 1574*

Speed, John, *Map of Cambridge, 1610*

Facsimiles published by Cambridgeshire Records Society, 2002

Unpublished Material

Wroth, R. 'Servants at St John's College, Cambridge', Advanced Diploma Dissertation, University of Cambridge, Institute of Continuing Education, 1998

Illustration Acknowledgements

Author's photograph, 10, 15, 19, 24, 29; Cambridgeshire Collection, Cambridge Central Library, 2, 5, 12, 14, 23, 26, 27; Cambridgeshire Record Society, 1, 6, 7; Newton Institute website, 16; Peter Mellows, 11; Syndics of Cambridge University Library, 8, 21, 30, 31; Wellcome Library, London, 3, 4, 18, 20, 22, 25, 28.

ACKNOWLEDGEMENTS

T HANKS ARE DUE to many people and institutions that have helped in the research and writing of this book. These include, in no particular order, the staff of the Cambridgeshire Archives and the Cambridgeshire Collection, staff of Cambridge University Library especially those in the Manuscript Room, Imaging Service and John Reynolds on the Issue Desk, whose advice on gardening is greatly missed now that he has retired. Numerous college archivists were unfailingly interested in the project and gave up their valuable time to help: Malcolm Underwood archivist of St John's College Cambridge, Geoffrey Thornton Martin archivist, Mrs Naomi Herbert and the staff of the Old Library Christ's College, Elizabeth Stratton, Edgar Bowring archivist of Clare College, and Robert Athol of the same college, Elizabeth Ennion-Smith archivist of St Catharine's College, Roger Lovatt archivist of Peterhouse, Frances Willmoth archivist of Jesus College, Kate Thompson archivist and Karen Lubarr librarian of Downing College. Thanks also go to Amelia Walker, senior library assistant of the Wellcome Library for her help in finding illustrations, to members of my family who sorted out computer problems, and to David Dymond who said that all history is about imagination when I was having doubts. Lastly and by no means least, thanks go to Heather McCallum, Rachael Lonsdale and Tami Halliday of Yale University Press for their input and encouragement.

Index